Perioperative Care

Editor

LORI S. WADDELL

VETERINARY CLINICS
OF NORTH AMERICA:
SMALL ANIMAL PRACTICE

www.vetsmall.theclinics.com

September 2015 • Volume 45 • Number 5

ELSEVIER

1600 John F. Kennedy Boulevard • Suite 1800 • Philadelphia, Pennsylvania, 19103-2899

http://www.vetsmall.theclinics.com

VETERINARY CLINICS OF NORTH AMERICA: SMALL ANIMAL PRACTICE Volume 45, Number 5

September 2015 ISSN 0195-5616, ISBN-13: 978-0-323-39125-2

Editor: Patrick Manley

Developmental Editor: Meredith Clinton

Veterinary Clinics of North America: Small Animal Practice (ISSN 0195-5616) is published bimonthly by Elsevier Inc., 360 Park Avenue South, New York, NY 10010-1710. Months of issue are January, March, May, July, September, and November. Business and Editorial Offices: 1600 John F. Kennedy Blvd., Ste. 1800, Philadelphia, PA 19103-2899. Customer Service Office: 3251 Riverport Lane, Maryland Heights, MO 63043. Periodicals postage paid at New York, NY and additional mailing offices. Subscription prices are $310.00 per year (domestic individuals), $500.00 per year (domestic institutions), $150.00 per year (domestic students/residents), $410.00 per year (Canadian individuals), $621.00 per year (Canadian institutions), $455.00 per year (international individuals), $621.00 per year (international institutions), and $220.00 per year (international and Canadian students/residents). To receive student/resident rate, orders must be accompanied by name of affiliated institution, date of term, and the *signature* of program/residency coordinator on institution letterhead. Orders will be billed at individual rate until proof of status is received. Foreign air speed delivery is included in all *Clinics* subscription prices. All prices are subject to change without notice. **POSTMASTER:** Send address changes to *Veterinary Clinics of North America: Small Animal Practice*, Elsevier Health Sciences Division, Subscription Customer Service, 3251 Riverport Lane, Maryland Heights, MO 63043. Customer Service (orders, claims, online, change of address): Elsevier Periodicals Customer Service, Elsevier Health Sciences Division Subscription **Customer Service 3251 Riverport Lane Maryland Heights, MO 63043. Tel: 1-800-654-2452 (U.S. and Canada); 314-447-8871 (outside U.S. and Canada). Fax: 314-447-8029. E-mail: journalscustomerservice-usa@elsevier.com (for print support); journalsonlinesupport-usa@elsevier.com (for online support).**

Reprints. For copies of 100 or more of articles in this publication, please contact the Commercial Reprints Department, Elsevier Inc., 360 Park Avenue South, New York, NY 10010-1710. Tel.: 212-633-3874; Fax: 212-633-3820; E-mail: reprints@elsevier.com.

Veterinary Clinics of North America: Small Animal Practice is also published in Japanese by Inter Zoo Publishing Co., Ltd., Aoyama Crystal-Bldg 5F, 3-5-12 Kitaaoyama, Minato-ku, Tokyo 107-0061, Japan.

Veterinary Clinics of North America: Small Animal Practice is covered in *Current Contents/Agriculture, Biology and Environmental Sciences, Science Citation Index, ASCA, MEDLINE/PubMed (Index Medicus), Excerpta Medica,* and *BIOSIS.*

Contributors

EDITOR

LORI S. WADDELL, DVM
Diplomate, American College of Veterinary Emergency and Critical Care; Adjunct Associate Professor, Critical Care, Intensive Care Unit, Department of Clinical Studies, Matthew J. Ryan Veterinary Hospital, University of Pennsylvania, School of Veterinary Medicine, Philadelphia, Pennsylvania

AUTHORS

INGRID M. BALSA, DVM
Department of Surgical and Radiological Sciences, University of California, Davis, Davis, California

LISA J. BAZZLE, DVM
Department of Small Animal Medicine and Surgery, College of Veterinary Medicine, University of Georgia, Athens, Georgia

KARI SANTORO BEER, DVM
Diplomate, American College of Veterinary Emergency and Critical Care; Lecturer, Critical Care, Intensive Care Unit, Department of Clinical Studies, Matthew J. Ryan Veterinary Hospital, University of Pennsylvania, School of Veterinary Medicine, Philadelphia, Pennsylvania

STEPHANIE H. BERRY, DVM, MS
Diplomate, American College of Veterinary Anesthesia and Analgesia; Assistant Professor, Department of Companion Animals, Atlantic Veterinary College, Charlottetown, Prince Edward Island, Canada

STUART BLISS, DVM, PhD
Diplomate, American College of Veterinary Surgeons; Port City Veterinary Referral Hospital, Portsmouth, New Hampshire

APRIL E. BLONG, DVM
Diplomate, American College of Veterinary Emergency and Critical Care; Department of Clinical Sciences, Cornell University College of Veterinary Medicine, Ithaca, New York

ELISE BOLLER, DVM
Diplomate, American College of Veterinary Emergency and Critical Care; Senior Lecturer, Emergency and Critical Care, Faculty of Veterinary and Agricultural Sciences, The University of Melbourne, Melbourne, Victoria, Australia

MANUEL BOLLER, Dr med vet, MTR
Diplomate, American College of Veterinary Emergency and Critical Care; Senior Lecturer, Emergency and Critical Care, Faculty of Veterinary and Agricultural Sciences, The University of Melbourne, Melbourne, Victoria, Australia

BENJAMIN M. BRAINARD, VMD
Diplomate, American College of Veterinary Anesthesia and Analgesia; Diplomate, American College of Veterinary Emergency and Critical Care; Department of Small Animal Medicine and Surgery, College of Veterinary Medicine, University of Georgia, Athens, Georgia

ANTHONY CARR, Dr med vet
Diplomate, American College of Veterinary Internal Medicine (Small Animal Internal Medicine); Professor, Department of Small Animal Clinical Sciences, Western College Veterinary Medicine, University of Saskatchewan, Saskatoon, Saskatchewan, Canada

STUART CLARK-PRICE, DVM, MS
Diplomate, American College of Veterinary Internal Medicine; Diplomate, American College of Veterinary Anesthesia and Analgesia; Assistant Professor of Anesthesia and Pain Management, Clinical Service Head, Anesthesia and Pain Management, Department of Veterinary Clinical Medicine, College of Veterinary Medicine, University of Illinois, Urbana, Illinois

WILLIAM T.N. CULP, VMD
Diplomate, American College of Veterinary Surgeons; Assistant Professor, Department of Surgical and Radiological Sciences, University of California, Davis, Davis, California

HAROLD DAVIS, BA, RVT, VTS (ECC) (Anesth)
Manager, Emergency and Critical Care Service, William R. Pritchard Veterinary Medical Teaching Hospital; School of Veterinary Medicine, University of California, Davis, Davis, California

TANYA DUKE-NOVAKOVSKI, BVetMed, MSc, DVA
Diplomate, American College of Veterinary Anesthesia and Analgesia; Diplomate, European College of Veterinary Anaesthesia and Analgesia; Professor of Veterinary Anesthesiology, Department of Small Animal Clinical Sciences, Western College Veterinary Medicine, University of Saskatchewan, Saskatoon, Saskatchewan, Canada

CHRISTOPHER W. FRYE, DVM
Department of Clinical Sciences, Cornell University College of Veterinary Medicine, Ithaca, New York

MARK A. OYAMA, DVM
Diplomate, American College of Veterinary Internal Medicine, Specialty of Cardiology; Department of Clinical Studies, Matthew J. Ryan Veterinary Hospital, University of Pennsylvania, School of Veterinary Medicine, Philadelphia, Pennsylvania

ELIZABETH A. ROZANSKI, DVM
Diplomate, American College of Veterinary Emergency and Critical Care; Diplomate, American College of Veterinary Internal Medicine (Small Animal Internal Medicine); Section of Critical Care, Cummings School of Veterinary Medicine, Tufts University, North Grafton, Massachusetts

LORI S. WADDELL, DVM
Diplomate, American College of Veterinary Emergency and Critical Care; Adjunct Associate Professor, Critical Care, Intensive Care Unit, Department of Clinical Studies, Matthew J. Ryan Veterinary Hospital, University of Pennsylvania, School of Veterinary Medicine, Philadelphia, Pennsylvania

JOSEPH J. WAKSHLAG, PhD, DVM
Diplomate, American College of Veterinary Nutrition; Diplomate, American College of
Veterinary Sports Medicine and Rehabilitation; Department of Clinical Sciences, Cornell
University College of Veterinary Medicine, Ithaca, New York

Contents

Perioperative patients can be highly dynamic and have various metabolic, physiologic, and organ system derangements that necessitate smart monitoring strategies and careful fluid therapy. The interplay between changing patient status, therapeutic interventions, and patient response makes effective monitoring crucial to successful treatment. Monitoring the perioperative patient and an approach to fluid therapy are discussed in this text.

Clinical assessment of tissue oxygenation is challenging. Anemia reflects a decreased oxygen carrying capacity of the blood and its significance in the perioperative setting relates largely to the associated risk of insufficient oxygen delivery and cellular hypoxia. Until meaningful clinical measures of tissue oxygenation are available in veterinary practice, clinicians must rely on evaluation of a patient's hemodynamic and ventilatory performance, along with biochemical and hemogasometric measurements. Blood transfusion is used commonly for treatment of perioperative anemia, and may improve tissue oxygenation by normalizing the rheologic properties of blood and enhancing perfusion, independent of increases in oxygen carrying capacity.

Perioperative complications commonly include oxygenation and ventilation abnormalities. The best outcome is associated with prevention. Ventilation impairment may be due to either neurologic compromise such as cervical intervertebral disk disease or severe parenchymal disease, while oxygenation failure may result from either the underlying disease or severe complications such as aspiration pneumonia, volume overload, pulmonary thromboembolism, or acute respiratory distress syndrome. This article reviews the approach to the patient with perioperative complications and provides recommendations on the management approach.

Obtaining and interpreting blood gas and electrolyte levels is essential in the management of perioperative veterinary patients. Metabolic and electrolyte alterations are common in critically ill surgical patients, and can lead to alterations in cardiovascular function, neurologic status, respiratory function, and even response to various drug therapies. Several common perioperative conditions are discussed in this article, including metabolic disturbances, electrolyte abnormalities (hyponatremia and hypernatremia, hyperkalemia), and respiratory abnormalities.

Perioperative disorders of heart rate and rhythm are common and can contribute to patient morbidity and mortality. Management of perioperative arrhythmias is facilitated by understanding the basic mechanisms of arrhythmia formation and the role of transient imbalances. The decisions of when and how to treat perioperative arrhythmias are based on whether or not hemodynamic signs are present and the assumed risk of sudden arrhythmic death. Perioperative arrhythmias warrant careful monitoring and consideration of potential complications associated with antiarrhythmic therapy.

Blood pressure monitoring and management is a vital part of the perianesthetic period. Disturbances in blood pressure, especially hypotension, can have significant impacts on the well-being of small animal patients. There are a variety of mechanisms present to control blood pressure, including ultra-short-, short-, and long-term-mechanisms. Several conditions can contribute to decreased blood pressure, including anesthetics, tension pneumothorax, intermittent positive pressure ventilation, hypoxemia, hypercapnia, surgical positioning, and abdominal distension. If hypotension is encountered, the initial response is to provide appropriate fluid therapy. If this is inadequate, other interventions can be used to increase blood pressure and thereby increase perfusion.

Inadvertent perianesthetic hypothermia is one of the most common complications in anesthesia of dogs and cats. Hypothermia during anesthesia can lead to altered pharmacokinetics of anesthetic and analgesic drugs, dysfunction of organ systems, increased patient susceptibility to infection, reduced wound healing, altered coagulation, hypotension, and delayed recovery. An understanding of the pathophysiology, complications, and techniques to minimize hypothermia during anesthesia can help veterinarians optimize care of patients. This article provides an overview of inadvertent perianesthetic hypothermia.

Although postoperative hemorrhage is an understood sequela, surgery also elicits an inflammatory response that may result in a hypercoagulable state and risk for venous or arterial thromboembolism. Postoperative venous thromboembolism is well documented in humans and is multifactorial in nature; however, evidence for its presence in veterinary medicine remains sparse. There is no consensus on the ideal type, dose, and duration of thromboprophylactic therapy in the perioperative period. Regardless, coagulation perturbations secondary to surgical stress are important considerations for the perioperative patient to reduce the possible fatal risks of hemorrhage or thrombosis.

Untreated or undermanaged perioperative pain has systemic effects that may negatively impact a patient's welfare and return to function. A consistent analgesic plan that assesses a patient's pain and comfort at regular intervals during the perioperative period should be incorporated into practice. Validated pain assessment tools are available for use in dogs and cats. Multimodal analgesic plans should be created for individual patients and modified according to pain assessments. These plans, based on a thorough history, physical examination, and knowledge of the expected pain, should be combinations of an opioid, a nonsteroidal anti-inflammatory drug, a local anesthetic, and nonpharmacologic analgesic techniques.

This article provides a general overview of nursing care principles including an approach to developing a nursing care plan using the nursing process as its foundation. The nursing process is a problem-solving approach used in planning patient care. This article also focuses on nursing care as it pertains to the respiratory, cardiovascular, and renal systems (fluid balance) as well as care of the recumbent patient. Knowledge of nursing care techniques and risk factors for complications puts the care provider in a position of being proactive rather than reactive to patient care needs.

Wound care requires an understanding of normal wound healing, causes of delays of wound healing, and the management of wounds. Every wound must be treated as an individual with regard to cause, chronicity, location, and level of microbial contamination, as well as patient factors that affect wound healing. Knowledge of wound care products available and when negative pressure wound therapy and drain placement is appropriate can improve outcomes with wound healing. Inappropriate product use

Peri-surgical nutrition of veterinary patients is in its infancy, with considerable research to be performed to help improve quality of life in our small animal patients. Clues from human immunonutrition may be starting places for investigation. Considerations for future investigations should include essential nutrients, the underlying disease process, therapeutic goals, and species (dog or cat). There are guidelines for caloric requirements. Planning for nutritional support before surgery takes place is likely to be beneficial to patient outcomes. Taking into account case history, method of feeding, metabolic abnormalities, and possible immunonutrition should be part of a complete surgical nutritional plan.

VETERINARY CLINICS OF NORTH AMERICA: SMALL ANIMAL PRACTICE

RELATED INTEREST

Veterinary Clinics of North America: Equine Practice
March 2015, Volume 31, Issue 1
Respiratory Medicine and Surgery
Sarah M. Reuss and A. Berkley Chesen, *Editors*

THE CLINICS ARE NOW AVAILABLE ONLINE!
Access your subscription at:
www.theclinics.com

Preface

Perioperative Monitoring

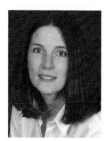

Lori S. Waddell, DVM
Editor

This issue of the *Veterinary Clinics of North America: Small Animal Practice* is dedicated to monitoring of the surgical patient: preoperatively, intraoperatively, and postoperatively. To maximize outcome in these patients, appropriate monitoring and care must be available. Even the most skilled surgeon would not have positive outcomes unless this essential care is provided.

Ideally, perioperative patients will have a highly skilled group of veterinarians caring for them. Throughout this issue, articles have been written by specialists in the fields of emergency and critical care, anesthesia, surgery, internal medicine, cardiology, veterinary nursing, and nutrition. This demonstrates the diverse knowledge from different areas of veterinary medicine that can be required for the treatment of the perioperative patient. Although such a team is not necessarily required for every patient, knowledge about all of these areas is essential for many, and this issue provides a valuable resource for the veterinarian that is working without such a team.

Management of the patient's volume status with fluid therapy, understanding the impacts of anemia and oxygen delivery, monitoring the respiratory system for appropriate oxygenation and ventilation, and the use of blood gases to monitor and treat acid-base and electrolyte disturbances are of paramount importance in these patients. Equally important are monitoring the cardiovascular system for abnormalities in blood pressure and heart rhythm, understanding the importance of thermoregulation and coagulation and their effects on the perioperative patient, knowing how to provide appropriate analgesia and nursing care, as well as optimizing wound healing, and providing appropriate nutrition for these patients. This issue focuses on these many aspects of care, with an article on each of these topics.

I would like to thank all of the authors that contributed to this issue of *Veterinary Clinics of North America: Small Animal Practice* for taking the time out of their busy clinic and teaching schedules. Together they have provided an excellent resource that will be used by veterinarians as they try to optimize the treatment of their surgical

Vet Clin Small Anim 45 (2015) xiii–xiv
http://dx.doi.org/10.1016/j.cvsm.2015.06.001
0195-5616/15/$ – see front matter © 2015 Published by Elsevier Inc.

patients. This information can improve the care of dogs and cats undergoing surgery. It provides a nice, concise summary of many of the aspects of perioperative monitoring that are utilized in the Emergency Service, Anesthesia, and Intensive Care Unit at the University of Pennsylvania Small Animal Hospital where I help care for many of the postoperative patients.

Lori S. Waddell, DVM
Intensive Care Unit
Department of Clinical Studies
Matthew J. Ryan Veterinary Hospital
University of Pennsylvania
School of Veterinary Medicine
3900 Spruce Street
Philadelphia, PA 19104, USA

E-mail address:
loriwadd@vet.upenn.edu

Assessment of Fluid Balance and the Approach to Fluid Therapy in the Perioperative Patient

CrossMark

Elise Boller, DVM*, Manuel Boller, Dr med vet, MTR

KEYWORDS

- Fluid therapy • Monitoring • Microcirculation • Goal-directed therapy
- Dog • Cat • Perfusion

KEY POINTS

- Perioperative patients constitute a heterogeneous population that can have various derangements that necessitate smart monitoring strategies and careful fluid therapy.
- The interplay between the patient and therapeutic interventions makes effective monitoring crucial to successful treatment.
- Global hemodynamic assessment is unlikely to give the clinician certainty about microcirculatory blood flow.
- It is reasonable to implement a goal-directed approach to resuscitation of perioperative veterinary patients that avoids positive fluid balance, but more prospective studies need to be done to evaluate the efficacy and safety of this approach.

INTRODUCTION

Perioperative patients can have various dynamic metabolic, physiologic, and organ system derangements that necessitate smart monitoring strategies and careful fluid therapy. These patients not only suffer the initial underlying insult, but also the subsequent "hits" that come along with that insult and with treatment (eg, periods of hypotension and hypoxemia, transfusion of blood products, anesthesia, tissue trauma associated with surgery). The clinician's role in treating these patients can be divided into the 3 phases of treatment, which, together, constitute the "perioperative period." The preoperative phase of treatment should focus on making the surgical patient a

The authors do not have any conflicts of interest to declare.
Emergency and Critical Care, Faculty of Veterinary and Agricultural Sciences, The University of Melbourne, 250 Princes Highway, Werribee, Melbourne, Victoria 3030, Australia
* Corresponding author.
E-mail address: elise.boller@unimelb.edu.au

Vet Clin Small Anim 45 (2015) 895–915
http://dx.doi.org/10.1016/j.cvsm.2015.04.011
0195-5616/15/$ – see front matter © 2015 Elsevier Inc. All rights reserved.
vetsmall.theclinics.com

suitable anesthetic candidate by optimizing perfusion and the balance between oxygen delivery and oxygen consumption and by correcting electrolyte and acid-base abnormalities. Intraoperatively can be even more challenging, because the patient's own capability to maintain circulatory homeostasis is severely impaired by the effects of anesthetics. Abnormalities of electrolyte and acid-base balance may continue intraoperatively. Postoperatively, the patient may have increased vascular permeability, low colloid osmotic pressure (COP), and be in a positive fluid balance. The heterogeneity of perioperative patients (eg, due to age, underlying disease processes, and surgical procedures), requires consideration in all phases of perioperative fluid management. This article describes a goal-directed approach to treatment of perioperative patients that uses upstream endpoints of resuscitation (the portion of the circulatory system that feeds the tissues), microcirculatory endpoints (the tissues themselves), and downstream endpoints (markers of the balance between oxygen delivery and consumption), as well as reviews body fluid balance and treatment options that are crucial to consider when treating perioperative patients.

THE IMPORTANCE OF MONITORING

The interplay between changing patient status, therapeutic interventions, and patient response makes effective monitoring crucial to successful treatment. Monitoring in the medical field refers to the process of retrieving data describing the physiologic status of a patient, often serially. The data can be continuous (eg, blood pressure), categorical (eg, mucous membrane color), or binary (eg, weight gain: yes/no), and the variables can be gathered at any time interval considered appropriate. As such, clinical monitoring serves at least 5 purposes (**Box 1**).

1. First, to aid in the therapeutic process by defining and recognizing *treatment endpoints* that should serve as the targeted goals of certain interventions. Consider a cat with hypoperfusion secondary to hypovolemic shock. Initial therapy may consist of acute resuscitative fluid therapy (ARFT) and the monitored variables may include mean arterial blood pressure and urine output.
2. Second, clinical monitoring serves to define and recognize *safety limits* applied to the therapeutic process, so as to minimize adverse events. To return to the example, ongoing ARFT will be harmful if the patient is unable to produce urine after volume repletion. Frequent urine output measurements will prevent this from happening unnoticed.
3. Third, *prognostic information* can be gained from single point measurements or changes in physiologic variables over time. For example, lactate clearance in response to initial resuscitative treatment of gastric dilation and volvulus can be prognostically useful.[1,2]

Box 1
Goals of patient monitoring

To know what treatment endpoints have been reached

To know that safety limits have been reached

To obtain prognostic information

To anticipate physiologic changes

To aid in the diagnostic process

---

4. Fourth, monitoring allows the clinician to *anticipate alterations* in the animal's condition early and thus address changes before they amount to a serious complication. For example, monitoring the gag reflex in a patient with neurologic disease or who is heavily sedated may prompt the clinician to protect the airway via intubation to avoid an aspiration event.
5. Finally, monitoring may aid in the *diagnostic* process. For example, respiratory distress in a cat that resolves after diuretic administration would suggest congestive heart failure as the cause; the monitored variables being respiratory rate, effort, and SpO_2.

FLUID BALANCE IN PERIOPERATIVE PATIENTS

Perioperative patients often receive large amounts of intravenous fluids to replenish an absolute or relative volume deficit. In the purest sense of the word, "dehydration" simply implies a fluid deficit from anywhere, clinically this term is used to describe an interstitial not intravascular deficit.

An understanding of total body water (TBW) and fluid compartments within the body is necessary to understand how body fluids shift in health and in states of disease. Total body water is approximately 60% of a normal adult animal's body weight and is divided into 2 major compartments: the intracellular fluid (ICF) and the extracellular fluid (ECF) spaces, which constitute two-thirds and one-third the TBW, respectively. These spaces are separated from each other by cell membranes that are permeable to water but impermeable to most solutes.

Within the ECF, the interstitial space refers to the space outside of the cells and outside of the vasculature, but includes lymph fluid; the interstitial space holds for approximately 75% of the ECF. A fluid loss in this compartment is generally referred to as "dehydration." The other portion of the ECF, the intravascular space, holds 25% of the ECF and contains the blood volume. This is the fluid space of primary concern when a patient is described as "hypovolemic." Patients can have various combinations of clinical fluid deficits or excesses in the intravascular and the interstitial spaces depending on the rate of fluid loss, the type of fluid lost, and vascular endothelial integrity. Importantly, the type of fluid lost (isotonic, hypotonic, or hypertonic) will dictate fluid movement between the ECF and ICF, such that osmolarity remains equilibrated between the 2 spaces.

Perioperative patients often have an overall reduction in TBW from a negative fluid balance to the extent that it affects tissue perfusion, but occasionally a perioperative patient may have a positive fluid balance. Perioperative patients and especially those with systemic inflammatory conditions (eg, after sepsis, major trauma, and burns) may suffer from increased microvascular permeability and low plasma oncotic pressure, hence are at risk of interstitial edema formation over the course of the perioperative period. Interstitial edema increases the radial diffusion distance for oxygen from the intramicrovascular space to the parenchymal cell and may thus critically reduce mitochondrial oxygen partial pressure. In addition to the obvious clinical manifestation of interstitial edema, other examples of pathologic edema and a positive fluid balance include noncardiogenic pulmonary edema (acute lung injury [ALI]/acute respiratory distress syndrome [ARDS]), intestinal edema, and myocardial edema; evidence suggests that perioperative ileus may in part be due to intestinal edema, and myocardial edema can contribute to cardiac dysfunction.[3,4] Moreover, lack of a positive fluid balance or even the occurrence of a negative fluid balance in perioperative patients was associated with improved outcomes in human clinical studies.[5–8] In a randomized controlled trial involving humans with ARDS, a strategy targeting a negative fluid balance while increasing COP by concurrent administration of furosemide and albumin improved oxygenation and hemodynamic stability.[9] Although not studied in veterinary patients, an approach that avoids positive fluid balance and attempts to normalize COP seems reasonable in both dogs and cats.

THE ROLE OF THE PHYSICAL EXAMINATION IN ASSESSING PERFUSION AND HYDRATION

A fundamental goal of resuscitation is to achieve sufficient tissue perfusion and substrate delivery to fulfill the metabolic needs of the tissue perfused. Physical examination (PE) parameters and smart longitudinal monitoring strategies are essential not only to gauge patient response to resuscitation but also to herald imminent fluid overload.

Clinical signs of hypoperfusion associated with hypovolemic, obstructive, or cardiogenic shock in dogs and cats are similar, despite differing etiologies. They include mental dullness due to decreased brain perfusion, tachycardia due to sympathoadrenergic stimulation, poor pulses because of decreased cardiac output (CO) and increased systemic vascular resistance (SVR), pale mucous membranes, prolonged capillary refill time (CRT) and cool extremities as an expression of peripheral vasoconstriction, and tachypnea, which is thought to be chemoreceptor mediated. With hypovolemic shock, these clinical signs of hypoperfusion follow a relatively predictable course as the loss of intravascular volume progresses (**Table 1**). Clinical signs of progressive interstitial dehydration have been well described elsewhere.[10] Severe, untreated dehydration in an animal without access to water or in one that is unable to drink will progress to circulatory shock secondary to intravascular volume depletion.

Clinical signs of hypoperfusion secondary to early distributive shock (eg, secondary to severe sepsis) in dogs include tachycardia, "bounding" or tall and wide pulses,

Table 1
Clinical examination parameters in progression hypoperfusion (hypovolemic)

Clinical Parameter	Mild Hypovolemia	Moderate Hypovolemia	Severe Hypovolemia
Heart rate, beats per minute	130–150 (dog)[a]	150–170 (dog)[a]	170–220 (dog)[a]
Mucous membrane color	Normal to hyperemic	Pale pink	Gray, white, or muddy
Capillary refill time	Rapid (<1 s)	1–2 s	Prolonged or absent >2 s
Femoral pulse pressure (amplitude)	Increased	Mild to moderately decreased	Severely decreased
Femoral pulse duration (width)	Mildly reduced (thin) – in combination with increased pulse pressure often called "snappy"	Moderately reduced	Severely reduced (in combination with reduced pulse pressure, often called "poor or thready")
Metatarsal pulse	Easily palpable	Just palpable	Absent, often with cold extremities

[a] Cats tend to have a less predictable heart rate response and can be tachycardic or bradycardic. When tachycardia occurs in cats, it tends to vary less from their normal heart rate as compared with dogs.

Adapted from Boag AK, Hughes D. Assessment and treatment of perfusion abnormalities in the emergency patient. Vet Clin North Am Small Anim Pract 2005;35(2):322; with permission.

hyperemic mucous membranes, tachypnea, warm extremities, and sometimes mental dullness. As distributive shock progresses from this initial hyperdynamic state, clinical signs gain in similarity to the other forms of shock described previously. In contrast to dogs, cats do not display the same hyperdynamic signs that dogs do with distributive shock, but rather, in the setting of sepsis, tend to be hypothermic, bradycardic, and hypotensive.[11]

Most of the previously mentioned PE parameters pertain to aspects of the circulation before the microcirculation (upstream parameters) or after the microcirculation (downstream parameters). Because the fundamental goal of resuscitation is aimed at satisfying the metabolic needs of the tissues, direct diagnostic examination of microcirculatory blood flow would be ideal. Mucous membrane color and CRT may be the only PE findings that assess the microcirculation. Advanced modalities for monitoring the microcirculation are described later in this article (see Direct assessment of the microcirculation).

Mentation and urine output can be considered clinical downstream endpoints of resuscitation that should be assessed in the perioperative patient. Urine output (UOP), normally greater than 2 mL/kg per hour, serves as an indirect measure for end-organ perfusion, is of great help with the management of fluid balance, and allows timely recognition of oliguria as a consequence of acute kidney injury should it occur.

Monitoring the global fluid balance by tracking the fluid volume administered and the volume eliminated by the animal in a quantitative fashion is "monitoring ins and outs." Doing so in a frequency adjusted to the animal's condition and in combination with serial body weights, UOP, urine specific gravity, central venous pressure (CVP), and mean arterial blood pressure (MAP), the clinician can fine-tune fluid and if needed, diuretic therapy to minimize the risk of inadvertent excessive positive or negative fluid balance. The use of worksheets to record ins and outs in 2-hour to 4-hour intervals allows trends to be tracked in fluid balance, so that appropriate adjustments to therapy can be made. To do this, a worksheet is designed to record volumes for "ins" (crystalloids, colloids, blood products, parenteral nutrition, bolused medications, and drugs given as continuous rate infusions) and "outs" (eg, UOP, vomiting, diarrhea, gastric residuals, cavitary effusions, outs from chest and abdominal drains) for a given time interval.

Monitoring of fluid balance by using patient body weight serially is another very useful parameter. The occurrence of generalized peripheral edema in dogs serves as an indicator of capillary leakage, and appears most prominently in the distal extremities, most noticeably around the hock, and dependant parts of the trunk and in the face, including the conjunctivae (although chemosis typically occurs only with moderate to severe edema). In cats, generalized overhydration is more diffusely distributed and therefore less obvious. Cats also have the tendency to form noncardiogenic pulmonary edema and pleural effusion at a relatively earlier stage then dogs, so overhydration has to be of particular concern in feline patients.

APPROACH TO FLUID THERAPY IN THE PERIOPERATIVE PATIENT

From a fluid balance perspective, there are 3 main indications for perioperative fluid therapy: to improve perfusion in the context of ARFT, to improve interstitial dehydration in the context of rehydration fluid therapy, and to provide for a patient's maintenance fluids and electrolyte needs at times when patients cannot or will not do so themselves. In addition to these commonly encountered fluid balance abnormalities, perioperative patients will also need monitoring and treatment of acid-base and electrolyte disturbances. When deciding on appropriate monitoring strategies, clinical decisions regarding the chosen approach to fluid therapy should include the following considerations:

- What is required: acute resuscitative, rehydration, or maintenance therapy, or a combination thereof?
- What fluids are available and what is the rationale for choosing a particular fluid?
- Does the patient have risk factors for developing complications of fluid therapy?

Acute Resuscitative, Rehydration, and Maintenance Fluid Therapy

Most patients will require some combination of concurrently administered acute resuscitative, rehydration, or maintenance fluid therapy over the course of the perioperative period. In hypoperfused patients, ARFT should be carried out immediately on recognition, whereas treatment for interstitial dehydration can occur over 4 to 24 hours. Perioperative patients who cannot or will not eat or drink require maintenance fluid therapy to supply metabolic water requirements. To design a fluid management plan for an individual patient, it is best to consider the need for each of these 3 basic categories of fluid therapy separately for the preoperative, intraoperative, and postoperative phases.

Acute resuscitative fluid therapy

ARFT is based on using aliquots of a blood volume sequentially, titrating to desired therapeutic goals, and safety limits. The blood volume in a dog is considered to be 80 to 90 mL/kg; in a cat it is estimated to be 60 mL/kg.[12] Depending on the severity of hypoperfusion and if there are risk factors present for developing complications of fluid therapy, a starting volume of an intravenous fluid is chosen. In dogs with uncomplicated moderate hypovolemia, 15 to 20 mL/kg of an isotonic crystalloid fluid can be administered over 10 to 15 minutes. If the severity of the shock is only mild or if there are risk factors present, the initial dose may be reduced to 10 to 15 mL/kg and given over 5 to 10 minutes. If the hypoperfusion is severe, the dose may be increased to 20 to 30 mL/kg. Doses should be adjusted downward for cats because of their smaller blood volume. Significant prolongation of the time over which the infusion is administered is not recommended, because rapid redistribution of crystalloid fluids occurs throughout the ECF. Thirty minutes after intravenous administration, only 25% of an isotonic crystalloid volume remains in the intravascular space.[13] Typically a balanced isotonic fluid such as lactated ringer solution (LRS) is used. However, there may be special circumstances that may lead to the preferential use of one crystalloid over another (see Perioperative Acid-Base and Electrolyte Disturbances by Drs Waddell and Santoro Beer, elsewhere in this issue).

Rehydration fluid therapy

A common approach to rehydration fluid therapy is to estimate the fluid deficit, decide over what period of time to correct it, and to administer the volume concurrently with maintenance fluid requirements. Additional ongoing losses are typically replaced as they occur. An approach to rehydration fluid therapy is summarized in **Table 2**. Balanced isotonic crystalloid fluids are typically used.

Maintenance fluid therapy

Maintenance fluid therapy involves administering fluids based on the animal's metabolic water requirements (**Box 2**). Several calculations for estimating maintenance fluid rates have been recommended,[14,15] and charts describing daily water and caloric requirements for the dog and cat are also freely available.[15]

Table 2	
Approach to rehydration fluid therapy	
1. Calculate the hydration deficit, divide by the number of hours over which it will be replaced (4–24 h)	Fluid deficit (mL) = estimated% dehydration as a decimal × body weight in kg × 1000
2. Calculate maintenance requirement	40–60 mL/kg/d
3. Replace ongoing losses (gastrointes-tinal, urinary, polyuria)	Measure every 4 h and replace over the following 4 h

Adapted from DiBartola SP, Bateman S. Introduction to fluid therapy. In: DiBartola SP, editor. Fluid, electrolyte, and acid-base disorders in small animal practice. 4th edition. Saint Louis (MO): W.B. Saunders; 2012. p. 348; and Muir WW, DiBartola SP. Fluid therapy. In: Kirk RW, editor. Current veterinary therapy VIII. Philadelphia: W.B. Saunders; 1983.

Preoperative Fluid Balance

Preoperatively, patients commonly have increased losses or decreased intake of fluid and therefore are often either hypoperfused, interstitially dehydrated, or both. Fluid losses in these patients may be sensible (urinary or gastrointestinal), insensible (respiratory), or both and may lead to an ECF deficit. Quite marked contraction of the ECF to the extent of overt shock may occur in patients with diarrhea and vomiting, and concurrent inability to eat and drink. Additionally, preoperative patients are typically fasted, which results in decreased fluid and electrolyte uptake from the gastrointestinal tract and further supports the occurrence of an ECF deficit. Preoperative patients also may experience loss of intravascular blood volume from hemorrhage (eg, trauma, coagulopathy, or neoplasia) leading to hypovolemic shock. Many preoperative patients will require *both* ARFT and rehydration therapy.

Intraoperative Fluid Balance

Intraoperatively, several factors will affect blood volume and tissue perfusion. Sensible and insensible losses continue, but the extent to which these types of losses occur during anesthesia is a topic of debate. Surgical patients are given drugs that affect vasomotor tone and CO. Additionally, the intraoperative period is associated with dampening of the expected sympathoadrenergic response to hypovolemia (either absolute or relative due to vasodilation associated with general anesthesia). The patient is therefore more reliant on interventions with fluids and drugs to maintain perfusion.

Intraoperative patients are typically given higher than maintenance rates (eg, 10 mL/kg per hour); however, there is evidence to suggest that this rate may be excessive under normal circumstances if the goal is to maintain a zero net balance for losses occurring during surgery other than from hemorrhage. To the contrary, this rate may be inadequate if the goal is to truly expand the intravascular space.[16] Most of the

Box 2
Maintenance requirement formulas
$70 \times$ (body weight in kg)$^{0.75}$
$30 \times$ (body weight in kg) $+ 70$
40 to 60 mL/kg/d
• Sensible losses (urine output): 27–40 mL/kg/d
• Insensible losses (fecal, cutaneous, respiratory): 13–20 mL/kg/d

crystalloids infused will rapidly redistribute throughout the ECF and it may stay there longer than normal in anesthetized patients due to lower urine production in the operative period,[17] thus to truly achieve and maintain expansion of the intravascular space, rates much higher than 10 mL/kg per hour would likely be needed. The collective clinical experience is that administering isotonic crystalloid fluids at 10 mL/kg per hour during anesthesia does not typically lead to adverse effects; however, the intraoperative fluid load and the consequent dilution of plasma proteins along with decreased UOP can contribute to a positive fluid balance and decreased COP postoperatively. Therefore, administration of colloids is often recommended when the goal is to achieve a more sustained expansion of the intravascular space or increase COP intraoperatively.[16] Pharmacologic intervention to correct the relative hypovolemia or decreased CO associated with general anesthesia is often indicated. Treatment with vasopressors or positive inotropes, respectively, can spare the patient from postoperative fluid overload, but one must ensure that an adequate circulating volume is available to circulate (see Perioperative Blood Pressure Control and Management by Drs Duke-Novakovski and Carr, elsewhere in this issue).

Postoperative Fluid Balance

Postoperative patients may have problems with maintaining intravascular volume due to increased losses, such as cavitary effusions, decreased water intake from ileus and anorexia, changes in blood composition from a decreased COP, or increased vascular permeability. Critically ill postoperative patients therefore require a carefully considered approach to fluid therapy with continuous monitoring of their fluid balance. This may involve selection of specialized fluids, such as plasma or synthetic colloids, or adjustment of sodium and water balance with carefully balanced fluid and diuretic therapy. Additionally, depending on the severity of illness of the patient, the postoperative period may be characterized by abnormalities of vasomotor tone and cardiac function and may therefore require vasopressors or positive inotropic medications. Optimizing fluid balance in postoperative patients can be the most challenging and yet the most rewarding phase of perioperative fluid therapy.

Intravenous Fluid Types

Broad categories of types of fluids include those containing electrolytes (crystalloids), those containing large molecules (colloids), and those composed primarily of water.

Crystalloid fluids can be balanced or nonbalanced, and can be isotonic, hypertonic, or hypotonic. Balanced (polyionic) solutions have an electrolyte composition that resembles that of the ECF, and isotonic solutions have a tonicity similar to that of the ECF. Examples of balanced crystalloids include LRS, Plasmalyte-148 and Normosol-R. Examples of isotonic crystalloids include 0.9% NaCl, Plasmalyte-148 and Normosol-R. Physiochemical characteristics of commonly used crystalloid solutions are outlined in **Table 3**.

Colloid solutions contain larger particles (colloids), water, and electrolytes. Colloids do not cross semipermeable membranes, namely the vascular membranes in health, and because they exert an osmotic pressure in the blood, they cause water to remain within the intravascular space. Colloid solutions are typically isotonic but they also can be formulated as hypertonic solutions. Colloid solutions can be broadly divided into synthetic and natural solutions. Dextrans, hydroxyethyl starches, polygelatins, cell-free hemoglobin solutions, and plasma are all colloid fluids.

The safety and efficacy of colloids have received considerable attention in the recent past. A recent meta-analysis of randomized controlled trials comparing the use of colloids to crystalloids in critically ill people requiring intravascular volume

Table 3
Physicochemical characteristics of various crystalloid solutions

Fluid	Osmolarity, mmol/L	Buffer, mEq/L	Sodium, mEq/mL	Chloride, mEq/mL	Potassium, mEq/mL	Calcium, mEq/mL	Magnesium, mEq/mL	Glucose, G/L
Normosol-R	296	Acetate 27 Gluconate 23	140	98	5	0	3	0
Plasmalyte-A	294	Acetate 27	140	98	5	0	3	0
LRS	272	Lactate 28	130	109	4	3	0	0
0.9% NaCl	308	None	154	154	0	0	0	0
5% dextrose in water	252	0	0	0	0	0	0	50
0.45% NaCl = 2.5% dextrose	280	None	77	77	0	0	0	25
3% NaCl	1026	0	513	513	0	0	0	0
7% NaCl	2567	0	1283	1283	0	0	0	0

Abbreviation: LRS, lactated ringer solution.

replacement showed that the use of colloids confers no advantage in reducing the risk of death compared with crystalloids.[18] In fact, this same systematic review called into question the safety of these fluids, with starches in particular possibly causing an increase in mortality. The Surviving Sepsis Campaign (2012 International guidelines for management of severe sepsis and septic shock) issued the avoidance of hetastarch formulations as one of its key recommendations.[19] There is no current compelling evidence in veterinary medicine to suggest strong recommendations for or against the use of colloids.[20]

Examples of solutions that contain mostly water are 5% dextrose in water and 2.5% dextrose in 0.45% NaCl. These solutions are not balanced but are isotonic until the dextrose is metabolized to water in vivo, and they are typically used to replace a free water deficit. Serum electrolyte and blood glucose concentrations must be closely monitored when using these solutions to avoid hyponatremia and hyperglycemia. Additionally, 0.45% NaCl is available. It is hypotonic because it does not contain dextrose and is also used to provide free water.

The indications for use of these 3 categories of fluids and their movement through the body fluid compartments differ. With ARFT, most of the volume of a crystalloid infused (70%) will redistribute throughout the ECF space in less than an hour, whereas colloids are retained within the intravascular space for longer.[13] Fluids that are relatively hypotonic compared with the patient's plasma will redistribute to the ICF. As such, to best prescribe appropriate fluid therapy, careful consideration should be given to patient characteristics, such as the types of deficit present, and therefore aim of therapy (intravascular, interstitial, or intracellular), other patient characteristics, such as changes in blood composition or vessel characteristics (hypoalbuminemia or vasculitis), and features of the fluid choices at hand.

Risk Factors for Developing Complications of Fluid Therapy

Risk factors for complications of fluid therapy should be considered when formulating a fluid therapy plan for perioperative patients (**Box 3**). Although these are not absolute contraindications, they demand to be taken into account when designing a fluid plan. Presence of risk factors should prompt the clinician to use monitoring strategies that use safety targets, for example, aiming for a CVP of no greater than 5 to 6 cm H_2O in a patient with known heart disease.

Box 3
Risk factors for developing complications of fluid therapy

Heart disease

Lung injury

Traumatic brain injury

Hemorrhage

Pathologic oliguria

Anuria

Hypoalbuminemia

Anemia

Severe sodium derangements

Hyperosmolar state

Vasculitis

RESUSCITATION ENDPOINTS AND GOAL-DIRECTED THERAPY

Resuscitation of the hemodynamically unstable perioperative patient ultimately targets optimization of tissue blood flow, such that tissue oxygen demand required for upholding both structural and functional integrity of cells and cell groups is met by appropriate oxygen delivery. Given the practical difficulty of directly quantifying microcirculatory function itself at the current state of technology, upstream and downstream markers are widely used as endpoints of resuscitation (**Fig. 1**). Importantly, neither MAP, CO, CVP, lactate, UOP, nor any other metric alone can independently serve as a single resuscitation endpoint. It is rather the integration of many of these parameters that together allow for the conclusion that a patient is fully resuscitated. Hence, standardization of care by defining single resuscitation endpoints is not necessarily appropriate and may be applicable only to very specific populations. A titrated approach individualizing the resuscitation effort based on clinical evaluation (mental status, mucous membrane color, CRT, heart rate, pulse quality, UOP), hemodynamic measurements (MAP, CO), and tissue oxygenation surrogates (lactate, central or mixed venous oxygen saturation $[S_vO_2/S_{cv}O_2]$, arteriovenous P_{CO_2} gradient) and, in the future, possibly direct observation of microcirculatory blood flow is more appropriate. This approach "bundles" groups of resuscitation endpoints such that the value of monitoring them singly is leveraged by monitoring them together.

In human medicine, there is widespread adoption of resuscitation strategies for both septic and perioperative patients that use targeting and monitoring of multiple tissue perfusion endpoints, known as early goal-directed therapy. A landmark randomized controlled trial published in 2001 by Rivers and colleagues[21] used a titrated approach

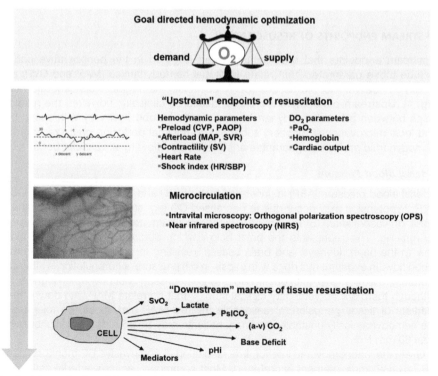

Fig. 1. Schematic describing the 3 levels on which resuscitation endpoints can be based.

to resuscitation in an early goal-directed algorithm for treatment of people with septic shock. In this study, resuscitation in the intervention group was started within 1 hour of admission to the emergency department. Parameters used as endpoints included arterial blood pressure (MAP $\geq$65 mm Hg and $\leq$90 mm Hg), CVP (8–12 mm Hg), and central venous oxygen saturation ($S_{cv}O_2$ $\geq$70%). The study showed a significant reduction in morbidity and improved survival rates in the intervention group. The tools used to reach these endpoints included crystalloid or colloid administration, vasoactive and inotropic agents, and red blood cell transfusions. Since then, multiple studies have supported these findings and revealed other benefits, such as modulation of inflammation, decreased organ failure, and conservation of health care resources.[22] Similar strategies in perioperative human patients have been studied and are advocated.[23–25]

There is limited but growing evidence that an early goal-directed approach may be beneficial to veterinary patients as well. In one study investigating changes in tissue perfusion parameters and outcome in dogs with severe sepsis/septic shock in response to goal-directed hemodynamic optimization, the investigators found that $S_{cv}O_2$, lactate, and base deficit on admission to the intensive care unit (ICU) were each independently associated with nonsurvival (P = .001, P = .030, and $P<.001$, respectively).[26] Additionally, $S_{cv}O_2$ and base deficit were found to be the best discriminators between survivors and nonsurvivors. The investigators concluded that $S_{cv}O_2$ and base deficit are useful in predicting the prognosis of dogs with severe sepsis and septic shock, and that animals with a higher $S_{cv}O_2$ and lower base deficit at admission to the ICU have a lower probability of death. The use of resuscitation endpoints, such as $S_{cv}O_2$ and base deficit in dogs with severe sepsis or septic shock may be prognostically useful, although few clinical studies have been published using such strategies in veterinary septic or perioperative patients.[27,28]

UPSTREAM ENDPOINTS OF RESUSCITATION

Upstream endpoints that are monitored and targeted in the perioperative patient include those parameters that relate to global hemodynamics (MAP and CVP) and to oxygen delivery to the tissues (DO_2), especially hemoglobin concentration (see **Fig. 1**). Upstream parameters are easily measured clinically; however, the relationships between global hemodynamics and regional blood flow vary with tissue bed and local microvascular function, such that no minimal perfusion pressure or global hemodynamic profile can guarantee adequate blood flow to all vascular beds.

Arterial Blood Pressure

Arterial blood pressure (ABP) is generated by both CO and SVR. Because BP = CO $\times$ SVR, hypotension may occur due to decreased CO (eg, stroke volume, heart rate, or both) or vasodilation (SVR). An often-cited minimum acceptable level of MAP is 60 mm Hg. This represents the point below which autoregulatory control of blood flow to the heart, kidneys, and brain ceases, resulting in pressure-dependent organ blood flow. In experimental dogs with sepsis, renal pressure-autoregulation is altered[29]; therefore, a MAP higher than 60 mm Hg may be necessary, but how much higher?[30,31] Although there are no veterinary clinical studies that correlate MAP with downstream markers of tissue perfusion, a reasonable minimal MAP that should be tolerated in the hemodynamically unstable veterinary patients may be 65 mm Hg or higher rather than 60 mm Hg.

Given the inaccuracy and inferior time resolution of noninvasive BP monitors, direct ABP (DABP) measurement is preferred. Most commonly, an intra-arterial catheter is placed into the dorsal pedal artery.[32]

Noninvasive or indirect blood pressure monitoring is accomplished via either Doppler sphygmomanometry or oscillometric blood pressure measurement. Both methods are less accurate than DABP measurement and do not provide the higher temporal resolution that DABP does. Only very few studies have compared gold standard (DABP) to noninvasive blood pressure (NIBP) modalities in hypotensive animals; the findings are varied but, generally speaking, measuring BP noninvasively is thought to be a clinically acceptable alternative to DABP monitoring. However, some of these studies showed decreased validity during periods of hypotension and increased difficulty in obtaining measurements when arrhythmias are present, particularly with oscillometric methods.[33–35]

Regardless of the chosen modality for measuring ABP, it cannot be stressed enough that BP considered in isolation is too crude of an endpoint to ensure adequate resuscitation in perioperative patients. In other words, hypotension generally indicates hemodynamic instability and is always of great concern, the reverse is not always true: normal ABP does not ensure cardiovascular stability.[16]

Shock Index

The value of measuring ABP may be increased by concurrently determining the shock index (SI), which is calculated by dividing heart rate by systolic BP (HR/SBP). It is a tool that is thought to be useful in identifying early shock, as routinely assessed cardiovascular parameters tend to remain within normal limits at that stage.[36] One veterinary study found a significant difference in SI between dogs with hemorrhagic shock and healthy controls.[37] Another study compared SI in healthy dogs, and dogs with and without shock presented to an emergency service.[38] This study also identified a significant difference in SI among these groups of dogs with animals in shock having a median SI significantly higher than those in the other 2 groups. This relatively simple clinical tool may be an additional valuable tool for assessing upstream parameters of perfusion, and emphasizes the diagnostic advantage of interpreting several hemodynamic variables in conjunction with each other.

Central Venous Blood Pressure

Monitoring CVP in the perioperative patient can be of twofold benefit. First, CVP serves as a safety endpoint, because the goal is ultimately to achieve hemodynamic optimization with the minimal hydrostatic pressure necessary. Second, CVP can be used in the dynamic process of a fluid challenge. Limiting hydrostatic pressure is of particular concern in critically ill perioperative patients, given the possibility of endothelial injury and the associated tendency for edema formation (both pulmonary and generalized). Pulmonary edema and respiratory failure (ALI/ARDS) are a real concern and constitute a major adverse event associated with ARFT, with cats are higher risk than dogs.

When using CVP monitoring, the tip of the central venous catheter is placed just outside the right atrium. During ventricular diastole, the tricuspid valve is open and the CVP is representative of right atrial filling pressure. The pressure obtained in this location is the hydrostatic pressure of the intrathoracic cranial vena cava, and is subject to pressure variations caused by other external forces, such as pleural space disease and positive pressure ventilation.

It must be noted that CVP monitoring as a static measure is an insensitive tool to predict fluid responsiveness.[39,40] Nevertheless, CVP can be used in the dynamic process of a fluid challenge to try to determine if the patient is fluid-responsive, specifically whether additional increases in right-sided filling pressures will result in any further increase in stroke volume or CO, or improve other global hemodynamic abnormalities, such as tachycardia or hypotension.[41,42]

A fluid challenge is performed by administering 10 to 15 mL/kg of an isotonic crystalloid fluid or 3 to 5 mL/kg of a colloid intravenously over 5 to 10 minutes followed by immediate reassessment of CVP along with MAP, HR, and so forth. If the endpoints are reached, the fluid challenge is discontinued. If the endpoint is not reached, the further process depends on the CVP alteration. The administration of fluid challenges continues until either the resuscitation endpoints are satisfied or the safety limits for filling pressures are reached (**Table 4**). Such an approach allows for a rapid sequence of small increments of fluid boluses in the face of clear endpoints, and therefore allows for fast and safe resuscitation. Although there are few data available in the literature with regard to what CVP is safe, clinical experience suggests that cats are more susceptible for pulmonary edema at a given CVP than dogs. Hence, a reasonable safety limit is a CVP of 5 cm H_2O in cats, and 10 cm H_2O in dogs. Maximally tolerated CVPs in the perioperative patient with sepsis or systemic inflammatory response syndrome may be lower than in the patient without a systemic inflammatory process.

Generally the issue with both the commonly used and the advanced "upstream modalities" (eg, transpulmonary thermodilution CO, lithium dilution CO, pulse contour analysis, partial carbon dioxide rebreathing, bioimpedance, and transesophageal echocardiography) is their distance from the actual tissues; observing the function of the microcirculation directly may provide valuable information with regard to both detecting and treating hemodynamically unstable patients. Indeed, there are numerous mechanisms by which microcirculatory function can be disturbed and advancing technologies by which this important aspect of tissue perfusion can be observed.

Although use of traditional and advanced upstream parameters is undoubtedly valuable, one cannot dismiss the potential disconnect between these parameters and the actual resultant flow to tissues. For example, studies directly visualizing sublingual microvascular blood flow found that vasodilators, like nitroglycerine, despite decreasing MAP, are capable of improving functional capillary density[43,44] even in disease processes characterized by low SVR such as sepsis. Given the vasodilatory effect of many drugs used during general anesthesia, a similar disconnect between global hemodynamic metrics and indices of microcirculatory function may exist. The same may be true when drugs such as α_2-agonists, which can produce intense

Table 4
Approach to using CVP to predict fluid responsiveness

Response to Fluid Challenge	Interpretation	Further Action
CVP rises <2 cm H_2O, or rises and quickly (<15 min) decreases again, does not rise	Hypovolemic: the patient may benefit by further fluid administration	Titrated small boluses to desired therapeutic target or safety limit
CVP rises 2–5 cm H_2O+/− returns toward baseline	Indeterminate (hypovolemic or euvolemic	Reevaluate in 10 min • If CVP has returned to patient baseline, repeat. • If CVP remains elevated discontinue challenge (euvolemia)
CVP rises >5 cm H_2O with slow return toward baseline (>30 min)	Euvolemic or hypervolemic (or reduced cardiac compliance)	Discontinue fluid challenge

Abbreviation: CVP, central venous pressure.

peripheral vasoconstriction, are used. Given the inability to directly assess the microcirculatory function currently, a downstream parameter like arterial lactate or $S_{cv}O_2$ should be used in addition to blood pressure.

DOWNSTREAM ENDPOINTS OF RESUSCITATION
Lactate

Using lactate as a downstream resuscitation endpoint is now considered standard of care in a multipronged approach to resuscitation of septic and perioperative human patients and is receiving significant attention in veterinary patients. In addition, analysis of serum lactate concentrations has gained recognition as an important prognosticator and useful diagnostic tool.

Lactate production serves as an important energy substrate when cellular energy requirements exceed aerobic energy production. Although serum lactate is useful to identify presence of tissue hypoxia, it is a late indicator of anaerobic metabolism. Thus, even a modest increase should be considered significant once other differentials for hyperlactatemia have been considered. One study evaluating lactate in hypotensive dogs found it to be negatively correlated with blood pressure and survival probability.[2] Another study evaluating goal-directed therapy and lactate in 8 critically ill dogs found that those animals whose serum lactate did not decrease by at least 50% during the first 6 hours of treatment were more likely to die.[45] In contrast, the lactate at time 0 as a static measurement had no prognostic significance in another study.[26] There are several other veterinary studies outlining its utility.[1,46–48] The information in both the human and veterinary literature strongly suggests 2 important points about lactate as an endpoint for resuscitation. First, lactate is a late indicator of energy debt and second, serial measurement rather than point is more powerfully prognostic.

There are several handheld lactate and bench-top analyzers available, and normal values may vary with the device used. A published lactate reference range for dogs aged 0.25 to 12 years was reported as 0.3 to 2.5 mmol/L.[49] A reasonable resuscitation endpoint for lactate would be a 50% reduction every 1 to 2 hours.[50]

Central and Mixed Venous Oxygen Saturation ($S_{cv}O_2/S_vO_2$)

Mixed venous oxygen saturation (S_vO_2) is measured in the pulmonary artery and hence reflects a weighted average of the oxygen saturation from venous blood originating from all parts of the body. The relationship between S_vO_2, CO, and whole body oxygen uptake (V_{O_2}) is described by the Fick principle in which the mixed venous oxygen content (C_vO_2) is calculated as follows:

$$C_vO_2 = C_aO_2 - (V_{O_2}/CO)$$

Hence, monitoring C_vO_2 (under the stipulation of constant C_aO_2) represents monitoring changes in the ratio of V_{O_2} and CO.

Mixed venous (C_vO_2) and arterial (C_aO_2) oxygen content are dependent on hemoglobin saturation (Hb), S_vO_2, and P_vO_2 and are expressed as follows:

$$C_vO_2 \text{ [mL/dL]} = (1.34[\text{mL/g}] \times (\text{Hb[g/dL]}) \times S_vO_2[\%]) + (0.003 \times P_vO_2[\text{mm Hg}])$$

$$C_aO_2 \text{ [mL/dL]} = (1.34[\text{mL/g}] \times (\text{Hb[g/dL]}) \times S_aO_2[\%]) + (0.003 \times P_aO_2[\text{mm Hg}])$$

Because the amount of dissolved oxygen as determined by P_vO_2 or P_aO_2 is a negligible quantity and because the hemoglobin concentration remains relatively stable over a certain period of time, S_vO_2 is the major variable contributing to C_vO_2. Under physiologic conditions, the oxygen extraction ratio is approximately 25%, thus a normal S_vO_2 is approximately 75% to 80%.[51]

By analyzing the formulas, it is clear that 4 single factors result in a decreased S_vO_2 (**Table 5**). Importantly, S_vO_2 can be pathologically increased in states of decreased Vo_2 (eg, cytopathic shock, hypoxia, microvascular shunting) or DO_2 (eg, increased CO in the hyperdynamic phase of septic shock).

Due to the difficulty in obtaining SvO_2, which requires placing a pulmonary artery catheter, $S_{cv}O_2$ (from blood from the vena cava on the level of the right atrium) has been measured as a surrogate for S_vO_2 in the clinical setting. As has been deducted from both human clinical and animal experimental studies, there is good correlation between central venous and mixed venous oxygen saturation under nonshock conditions, whereas in most shock settings, the exact correlation between the 2 is a matter of controversy. However, in standardized bundle resuscitation in people it is now widely accepted to use $S_{cv}O_2$.[19] Treatment decisions should primarily be based on response to intervention and trends. Human data suggest that outcome can be improved when $S_{cv}O_2$ of greater than 70% is targeted as a resuscitation endpoint.[23,25,52] Higher $S_{cv}O_2$ and a lower base deficit at admission to the ICU was associated with a lower probability of death in dogs with severe sepsis/septic shock and a higher risk of death was identified in critically ill dogs with a $S_{cv}O_2$ of less than 68%.[26,53]

The current literature suggests that a significant oxygen debt occurs perioperatively and, in particular, postoperatively. Studies demonstrate a sharp decline in $S_{cv}O_2$ and S_vO_2 immediately after surgery and that the degree of oxygen debt is significantly correlated with postoperative complications such as acute kidney injury, infections, myocardial ischemia, and death.[54] The current recommendation for the intraoperative and postoperative periods is to maintain $S_{cv}O_2$ above 70%. For instance, an $S_{cv}O_2$ value of 60% would warrant further fluid administration, the use of a positive inotrope, like dobutamine, judicious use of a vasopressor, or in case of a decreased hemoglobin concentration, transfusion of red blood cells. This approach requires intensive care monitoring in the 8-hour to 12-hour postoperative period. Importantly, $S_{cv}O_2$ greater than 70% does not guarantee absence of an imbalance between oxygen consumption and oxygen delivery, given the potential for cytopathic hypoxia and microvascular shunting in sepsis. By the same token, a patient that appears hemodynamically stable by traditional measures (eg, mentation, heart rate, pulse quality, BP) may experience significant tissue hypoperfusion and oxygen debt.[55]

Because placement of a central venous catheter is warranted and feasible in many sick perioperative dogs and cats, $S_{cv}O_2$ measurements could be incorporated into the monitoring plan. $S_{cv}O_2$ can be determined using blood gas analyzers, co-oximetry, or

Table 5
Factors contributing to decreased S_vO_2

Factors	Treatment
1. Arterial hypoxemia (decreased S_aO_2)	Supplemental oxygen, ventilation
2. Increased oxygen consumption (Vo_2) in the face of normal C_aO_2 and CO	Decrease the work of breathing (ie, mechanical ventilation), treating fever or hyperthermia
3. Decreased CO	Inotropic support, fluids
4. Decreased hemoglobin	Red blood cell transfusions

Abbreviation: CO, cardiac output.

continuous spectrophotometry. When using a blood gas analyzer for measuring $S_{cv}O_2$, a blood sample has to be taken each time leading to increased cost and blood loss. Contraindications are few and relate to jugular catheter placement.

Venoarterial CO_2 Gradient

Tissue hypoperfusion can result in tissue hypercapnia. The gradient between the arterial and venous CO_2 describes the relationship among ventilation, tissue CO_2 production, and pulmonary blood flow. Assuming constant ventilation (Pa_{CO_2}), even when tissue CO_2 production remains constant, sluggish microcirculatory blood flow can result in venous hypercapnia. This results in a widened gap between arterial and venous P_{CO_2} (Pa-vCO_2 gradient). Pa-vCO_2 has been used as a downstream marker for tissue hypoperfusion similar to lactate; combining these 2 downstream parameters was shown to increase the sensitivity for detecting tissue hypoperfusion in human perioperative patients and in dogs with experimental cardiac tamponade.[56,57] Like all other monitoring modalities, Pa-vCO_2 by itself and/or as a static measurement is not likely to provide the higher resolution information that one gets by combining modalities and trending values over time.

DIRECT ASSESSMENT OF THE MICROCIRCULATION

Assessment, monitoring, and protection of the microcirculation is currently a hot topic of investigation. It is likely that direct visualization techniques, such as sidestream darkfield imaging (**Fig. 2**), and other indirect measures, such as tissue P_{CO_2} and monitoring microvascular reactivity using near-infrared spectroscopy, may emerge as clinically useful tools in the future.[58,59]

CURRENT CONTROVERSIES AND FUTURE CONSIDERATIONS

The assessment and care of perioperative veterinary patients is an issue that veterinarians in most clinical contexts face daily. Future challenges include further defining knowledge gaps in the area of assessment of fluid balance and fluid therapy in veterinary patients; refining goal-directed therapy for our patients with prospective clinical studies; developing an understanding of the role and safety of colloids in dogs and

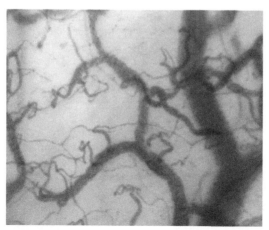

Fig. 2. Example of an image of the sublingual microcirculation, acquired using a sidestream dark field imaging system.

cats; developing strategies for reconciling the gap between assessments of global hemodynamics with that of the microcirculation; and developing and implementing practical tools for the assessment of microcirculation.

SUMMARY

Perioperative patients constitute a heterogeneous population that can have various metabolic, physiologic, and organ system derangements that necessitate smart monitoring strategies and careful fluid therapy. The interplay between changing patient status, therapeutic interventions, and patient response makes effective monitoring crucial to successful treatment. Because regulatory events act at several levels in both macrovascular and microvascular domains to affect tissue perfusion, global hemodynamic assessment is unlikely to give the clinician certainty about microcirculatory blood flow. It is reasonable to implement a goal-directed approach to resuscitation of perioperative veterinary patients that avoids positive fluid balance, but more prospective studies need to be done to evaluate the efficacy and safety of this approach.

REFERENCES

1. Zacher LA, Berg J, Shaw SP, et al. Association between outcome and changes in plasma lactate concentration during presurgical treatment in dogs with gastric dilatation-volvulus: 64 cases (2002-2008). J Am Vet Med Assoc 2010;236:892–7.
2. Ateca LB, Dombrowski SC, Silverstein DC. Survival analysis of critically ill dogs with hypotension with or without hyperlactatemia: 67 cases (2006-2011). J Am Vet Med Assoc 2015;246:100–4.
3. Bijnens B, Sutherland GR. Myocardial oedema: a forgotten entity essential to the understanding of regional function after ischaemia or reperfusion injury. Heart 2008;94:1117–9.
4. Uray KS, Laine GA, Xue H, et al. Intestinal edema decreases intestinal contractile activity via decreased myosin light chain phosphorylation. Crit Care Med 2006; 34:2630–7.
5. Bundgaard-Nielsen M, Secher NH, Kehlet H. 'Liberal' vs. 'restrictive' perioperative fluid therapy—a critical assessment of the evidence: review article. Acta Anaesthesiol Scand 2009;53:843–51.
6. Barmparas G, Liou D, Lee D, et al. Impact of positive fluid balance on critically ill surgical patients: a prospective observational study. J Crit Care 2014;29:936–41.
7. Alsous F, Khamiees M, DeGirolamo A, et al. Negative fluid balance predicts survival in patients with septic shock: a retrospective pilot study. Chest 2000;117: 1749–54.
8. Boyd JH, Forbes J, Nakada TA, et al. Fluid resuscitation in septic shock: a positive fluid balance and elevated central venous pressure are associated with increased mortality. Crit Care Med 2011;39:259–65.
9. Martin GS, Moss M, Wheeler AP, et al. A randomized, controlled trial of furosemide with or without albumin in hypoproteinemic patients with acute lung injury. Crit Care Med 2005;33:1681–7.
10. Mathews KA. Chapter 16-Monitoring fluid therapy and complications of fluid therapy. In: DiBartola SP, editor. Fluid, electrolyte, and acid-base disorders in small animal practice. 4th edition. Saint Louis (MO): W.B. Saunders; 2012. p. 386–404.
11. Costello MF, Drobatz KJ, Aronson LR, et al. Underlying cause, pathophysiologic abnormalities, and response to treatment in cats with septic peritonitis: 51 cases (1990-2001). J Am Vet Med Assoc 2004;225:897–902.

12. Wellman ML, DiBartola SP, Kohn CW. Chapter 1-Applied physiology of body fluids in dogs and cats. In: DiBartola SP, editor. Fluid, electrolyte, and acid-base disorders in small animal practice. 4th edition. Saint Louis (MO): W.B. Saunders; 2012. p. 2–25.

13. Silverstein DC, Aldrich J, Haskins SC, et al. Assessment of changes in blood volume in response to resuscitative fluid administration in dogs. J Vet Emerg Crit Care 2005;15:185–92.

14. O'Toole E, Miller CW, Wilson BA, et al. Comparison of the standard predictive equation for calculation of resting energy expenditure with indirect calorimetry in hospitalized and healthy dogs. J Am Vet Med Assoc 2004;225:58–64.

15. DiBartola SP, Bateman S. Chapter 14-Introduction to fluid therapy. In: DiBartola SP, editor. Fluid, electrolyte, and acid-base disorders in small animal practice. 4th edition. Saint Louis (MO): W.B. Saunders; 2012. p. 331–50.

16. Pascoe PJ. Chapter 17-Perioperative management of fluid therapy. In: DiBartola SP, editor. Fluid, electrolyte, and acid-base disorders in small animal practice. 4th edition. Saint Louis (MO): W.B. Saunders; 2012. p. 405–35.

17. Boscan P, Pypendop BH, Siao KT, et al. Fluid balance, glomerular filtration rate, and urine output in dogs anesthetized for an orthopedic surgical procedure. Am J Vet Res 2010;71:501–7.

18. Perel P, Roberts I, Ker K. Colloids versus crystalloids for fluid resuscitation in critically ill patients. Cochrane database Syst Rev 2013;(2):CD000567.

19. Dellinger RP, Levy MM, Rhodes A, et al. Surviving sepsis campaign: international guidelines for management of severe sepsis and septic shock: 2012. Crit Care Med 2013;41:580–637.

20. Adamik KN, Yozova ID, Regenscheit N. Controversies in the use of hydroxyethyl starch solutions in small animal emergency and critical care. J Vet Emerg Crit Care 2015;25:20–47.

21. Rivers E, Nguyen B, Havstad S, et al. Early goal-directed therapy in the treatment of severe sepsis and septic shock. N Engl J Med 2001;345:1368–77.

22. Rivers EP, Katranji M, Jaehne KA, et al. Early interventions in severe sepsis and septic shock: a review of the evidence one decade later. Minerva Anestesiol 2012;78:712–24.

23. Marik PE. Perioperative hemodynamic optimization: a revised approach. J Clin Anesth 2014;26:500–5.

24. Dalfino L, Giglio MT, Puntillo F, et al. Haemodynamic goal-directed therapy and postoperative infections: earlier is better. A systematic review and meta-analysis. Crit Care 2011;15:R154.

25. Cecconi M, Corredor C, Arulkumaran N, et al. Goal directed therapy: what is the evidence in surgical patients? Crit Care 2012;17(2):209.

26. Conti-Patara A, de Araujo Caldeira J, de Mattos-Junior E, et al. Changes in tissue perfusion parameters in dogs with severe sepsis/septic shock in response to goal-directed hemodynamic optimization at admission to ICU and the relation to outcome. J Vet Emerg Crit Care (San Antonio) 2012;22:409–18.

27. Prittie J. Optimal endpoints of resuscitation and early goal-directed therapy. J Vet Emerg Crit Care 2006;16:329–39.

28. Butler AL. Goal-directed therapy in small animal critical illness. Vet Clin North Am Small Anim Pract 2011;41:817–38, vii.

29. Yang R, Wang X, Liu S, et al. Changes of renal hemodynamics in dogs with endotoxemic shock. Zhonghua Yi Xue Za Zhi 2014;94:223–6 [in Chinese].

30. LeDoux D, Astiz ME, Carpati CM, et al. Effects of perfusion pressure on tissue perfusion in septic shock. Crit Care Med 2000;28:2729–32.

31. Thooft A, Favory R, Salgado DR, et al. Effects of changes in arterial pressure on organ perfusion during septic shock. Crit Care 2011;15:R222.
32. Silverstein D, Hopper K. Small animal critical care medicine. 2nd edition. St Louis (MO): Elsevier Saunders; 2015.
33. Bosiack AP, Mann FA, Dodam JR, et al. Comparison of ultrasonic Doppler flow monitor, oscillometric, and direct arterial blood pressure measurements in ill dogs. J Vet Emerg Crit Care 2010;20:207–15.
34. Shih A, Robertson S, Vigani A, et al. Evaluation of an indirect oscillometric blood pressure monitor in normotensive and hypotensive anesthetized dogs. J Vet Emerg Crit Care 2010;20:313–8.
35. Drynan EA, Raisis AL. Comparison of invasive versus noninvasive blood pressure measurements before and after hemorrhage in anesthetized greyhounds using the Surgivet V9203. J Vet Emerg Crit Care 2013;23:523–31.
36. Chan DL. Triage 2.0: re-evaluation of early patient assessment. J Vet Emerg Crit Care 2013;23:487–8.
37. Peterson KL, Hardy BT, Hall K. Assessment of shock index in healthy dogs and dogs in hemorrhagic shock. J Vet Emerg Crit Care 2013;23:545–50.
38. Porter AE, Rozanski EA, Sharp CR, et al. Evaluation of the shock index in dogs presenting as emergencies. J Vet Emerg Crit Care 2013;23:538–44.
39. Coudray A, Romand JA, Treggiari M, et al. Fluid responsiveness in spontaneously breathing patients: a review of indexes used in intensive care. Crit Care Med 2005;33:2757–62.
40. Marik PE, Baram M, Vahid B. Does central venous pressure predict fluid responsiveness? A systematic review of the literature and the tale of seven mares. Chest 2008;134:172–8.
41. Weil MH, Henning RJ. New concepts in the diagnosis and fluid treatment of circulatory shock. Anesth Analg 1979;58:124–32.
42. Vincent JL, Weil MH. Fluid challenge revisited. Crit Care Med 2006;34:1333–7.
43. Spronk PE, Ince C, Gardien MJ, et al. Nitroglycerin in septic shock after intravascular volume resuscitation. Lancet 2002;360:1395–6.
44. Lima A, van Genderen ME, van Bommel J, et al. Nitroglycerin reverts clinical manifestations of poor peripheral perfusion in patients with circulatory shock. Crit Care 2014;18:R126.
45. Stevenson CK, Kidney BA, Duke T, et al. Serial blood lactate concentrations in systemically ill dogs. Vet Clin Pathol 2007;36:234–9.
46. Sharkey LC, Wellman ML. Use of lactate in small animal clinical practice. Vet Clin North Am Small Anim Pract 2013;43:1287–97.
47. Mooney E, Raw C, Hughes D. Plasma lactate concentration as a prognostic biomarker in dogs with gastric dilation and volvulus. Top Companion Anim Med 2014;29:71–6.
48. De Papp E, Drobatz KJ, Hughes D. Plasma lactate concentration as a predictor of gastric necrosis and survival among dogs with gastric dilatation-volvulus: 102 cases (1995-1998). J Am Vet Med Assoc 1999;215:49–52.
49. Hughes D, Rozanski ER, Shofer FS, et al. Effect of sampling site, repeated sampling, pH, and Pco2 on plasma lactate concentration in healthy dogs. Am J Vet Res 1999;60:521–4.
50. Rosenstein PG, Hughes D. Hyperlactatemia. In: Silverstein D, Hopper K, editors. Small animal critical care medicine. 2nd edition. St Louis (MO): Elseveir Saunders; 2015. p. 300–5.
51. Haskins S, Pascoe PJ, Ilkiw JE, et al. Reference cardiopulmonary values in normal dogs. Comp Med 2005;55:156–61.

52. Rivers EP, Ahrens T. Improving outcomes for severe sepsis and septic shock: tools for early identification of at-risk patients and treatment protocol implementation. Crit Care Clin 2008;24:S1–47.
53. Hayes GM, Mathews K, Boston S, et al. Low central venous oxygen saturation is associated with increased mortality in critically ill dogs. J Small Anim Pract 2011; 52:433–40.
54. Bracht H, Eigenmann V, Haenggi M, et al. Multicentre study on peri- and postoperative central venous oxygen saturation in high-risk surgical patients. Crit Care 2006;10:R158.
55. Young BC, Prittie JE, Fox P, et al. Decreased central venous oxygen saturation despite normalization of heart rate and blood pressure post shock resuscitation in sick dogs. J Vet Emerg Crit Care (San Antonio) 2014;24:154–61.
56. Zhang H, Vincent JL. Arteriovenous differences in PCO2 and pH are good indicators of critical hypoperfusion. Am Rev Respir Dis 1993;148:867–71.
57. Silva JM, Oliveira AM, Segura JL, et al. A large venous-arterial PCO2 is associated with poor outcomes in surgical patients. Anesthesiol Res Pract 2011;2011: 759792.
58. De Backer D, Donadello K, Cortes DO. Monitoring the microcirculation. J Clin Monit Comput 2012;26:361–6.
59. Boag A, Hughes D. Assessment and treatment of perfusion abnormalities in the emergency patient. In: Assessment and treatment of perfusion abnormalities in the emergency patient. Philadelphia: Elsevier; 2005. p. 319.

Anemia and Oxygen Delivery

Stuart Bliss, DVM, PhD

KEYWORDS

- Anemia • Hematocrit • Hemoglobin • Perfusion • Viscosity

KEY POINTS

- Tissue oxygenation requires both adequate oxygen delivery and effective microvascular perfusion.
- The effects of perioperative anemia cannot be accurately assessed until normovolemia is established.
- The oxygen debt that occurs in severe anemia is caused in part by compromised microvascular blood flow associated with reductions in blood viscosity.
- Blood transfusion can improve tissue oxygenation by normalizing blood viscosity and restoring capillary perfusion as well as by augmenting oxygen carrying capacity.

INTRODUCTION

Oxygen delivery involves the unidirectional transport of oxygen from the atmosphere to the interior of the mitochondria within all of the body's cells. Red blood cells (RBCs) play a dominant role in the convective transport of oxygen from the lungs to the microvasculature. Anemia is a common comorbidity in surgical patients that can complicate perioperative care by compromising oxygen delivery and leading to tissue hypoxia. This article focuses on the effects of anemia on oxygen delivery. Quantitative aspects of global oxygen delivery and the role of hemoglobin (Hb) in gas transport are reviewed. Key concepts regarding microvascular blood flow and its impact on regional oxygen delivery are discussed. Physiologic effects of anemia are summarized. In addition, clinical assessment and management of anemia in the perioperative period are touched on from the perspective of microvascular function.

DETERMINANTS OF TISSUE OXYGENATION

Global oxygen delivery can be described quantitatively by the following familiar equations:

$$Do_2 = CO \times Cao_2 \tag{1}$$

Conflicts of interest: The author declares that there are no financial conflicts of interest.
Port City Veterinary Referral Hospital, 215 Commerce Way, Portsmouth, NH 03801, USA
E-mail address: sbliss@ivghospitals.com

where Do_2 is whole-body oxygen delivery, CO is cardiac output, and Cao_2 is the oxygen content within arterial blood. Under physiologic condition, 1 g of saturated Hb binds approximately 1.34 mL of oxygen. Cao_2 can therefore be calculated as:

$$Cao_2 \text{ (in mL/dL)} = [Hb](g/dL) \times 1.34 \text{ (mL/g)} \times Sao_2 + (0.003 \times Pao_2) \tag{2}$$

where $[Hb](g/dL)$ is the blood Hb concentration in grams per deciliter, Sao_2 is the percent saturation of Hb, 0.003 is the solubility coefficient of oxygen in plasma, and Pao_2 is the partial pressure of oxygen in the arterial blood. For animals breathing room air, dissolved oxygen accounts for approximately 2% of Cao_2, and its contribution is often disregarded. Thus, Cao_2 can be approximated as:

$$Cao_2 \text{ (mL/dL)} = [Hb](g/dL) \times 1.39 \text{ (mL/g)} \times Sao_2 \tag{3}$$

However, for animals receiving oxygen supplementation, dissolved oxygen can make up a significant proportion of overall delivered oxygen. This point is discussed in more detail later.

The amount of oxygen consumed by the body is expressed as:

$$Vo_2 = CO \times (Cao_2 - Cvo_2) \tag{4}$$

where Vo_2 is total oxygen consumption, and Cvo_2 is the oxygen content within the mixed venous blood of the main pulmonary artery. The fraction of delivered oxygen that is used by the body is the oxygen extraction ratio (o_2ER), expressed as:

$$o_2ER = Vo_2/Do_2 \tag{5}$$

Rearranging Equation 5 and substituting yields the following:

$$Vo_2 = CO \times [Hb](g/dL) \times 1.34 \times Sao_2 \times o_2ER \tag{6}$$

Equation 6 expresses the relationship between oxygen consumption and the parameters that determine oxygen delivery. For a given rate of Vo_2, a decrease in any of the parameters on the right of Equation 6 must be matched by a reciprocal change in 1 or more of the other parameters. Likewise, an increase in oxygen demand (Vo_2) can only be met by a proportional increase in 1 or more of the terms on the opposite side of the equation. Although Equation 6 refers to whole-body Vo_2, it is easy to appreciate how this basic relationship can be used to describe the balance between Vo_2 and Do_2 on regional, organ-specific, or even microvascular scales, by substituting tissue-specific blood flow for CO.

Normal o_2ER is approximately 25%; that is, the amount of oxygen delivered to the body exceeds overall tissue requirements by a factor of approximately 4.[1] A prominent exception is the myocardium, which consumes approximately 50% of delivered oxygen. The excess of Do_2 in relation to Vo_2 represents the physiologic reserve in Do_2 capacity, and is an evolutionary adaptation that ensures adequate oxygen supply to tissues despite moment-to-moment fluctuations in Do_2. As such, the relationship between Do_2 and Vo_2 is biphasic (**Fig. 1**). The upper portion of the curve represents the supply-independent region, where physiologic reserves and compensatory responses maintain Vo_2 despite a decrease in Do_2. However, below a threshold value of Do_2, termed the anaerobic threshold, compensatory mechanisms become exhausted, and Vo_2 becomes limited by Do_2 (supply dependency). The value of Do_2 corresponding with the anaerobic threshold is the Do_2crit, representing the critical level of oxygen delivery below which tissue hypoxia develops.

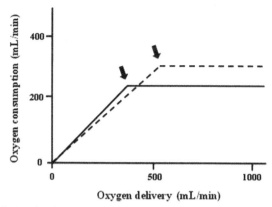

Fig. 1. Biphasic relationship between oxygen delivery and consumption. The horizontal portions of the curves represent the supply-independent phase, in which compensatory mechanisms maintain constant oxygen consumption despite decreased delivery. Below the anaerobic threshold (*arrows*), consumption becomes limited by delivery and tissue hypoxia develops. The dashed line represents a hypothetical Vo_2-Do_2 relationship for a postsurgical patient with increased oxygen demand and increased Do_2 crit (the critical level of oxygen delivery below which tissue hypoxia develops). (*Data from* Hebert J, Hu LQ, Biro G. Review of physiologic mechanisms in response to anemia. Can Med Assoc J 1997;156:S27–39.)

HEMOGLOBIN

Hb is the molecular vehicle responsible for transport of oxygen from the lungs to the tissues. Hb is a tetrameric protein complex consisting of symmetrically paired polypeptide heterodimers, each made up of alpha and beta globin subunits. Each globin molecule contains a non–covalently bound heme unit with a single iron atom. Under normal conditions, a small proportion of Hb exists as either methemoglobin or carboxyhemoglobin, neither of which is capable of binding oxygen. The association of oxygen with Hb is finely regulated through interactions with other molecules, such as protons, organic anions, and 2,3-bisphosphoglycerate (2,3-BPG).[2]

Desaturated Hb has a low affinity for oxygen; however, the initial binding of a single oxygen molecule increases the oxygen affinity of the Hb complex and facilitates additional oxygen binding. These properties are caused by allosteric changes in the Hb tetramer. Likewise, although fully saturated Hb maintains a high affinity for oxygen, dissociation of 1 oxygen molecule decreases overall oxygen affinity and promotes additional oxygen off-loading. This cooperativity in oxygen binding underlies the efficiency of Hb as an oxygen carrier, because it facilitates both oxygen uptake in the lungs and off-loading in the microvasculature. Cooperative oxygen binding is reflected in the sigmoidal shape of the familiar oxyhemoglobin dissociation curve (**Fig. 2**).

Hb also functions as a carrier of 3 other gases: carbon monoxide, carbon dioxide (CO_2), and nitric oxide (NO). Carbon monoxide binds with high affinity to the heme iron of Hb in competition with oxygen. Small amounts of carbon monoxide are produced endogenously as a product of heme degradation, and there is growing interest in the physiologic roles of carbon monoxide as a signaling molecule with cytoprotective and antiinflammatory properties.[3] CO_2 is transported primarily in solution in the plasma; however, some CO_2 may be transported by Hb through low-affinity interactions with amino-terminal residues of globin subunits.[4] NO is a gaseous free radical with potent vasodilatory properties that is produced by endothelial cells and RBCs.[5] NO can react with oxyhemoglobin to produce methemoglobin and nitrate ions, a

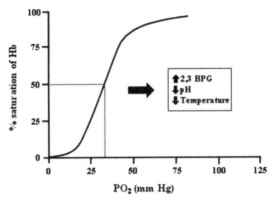

Fig. 2. The oxyhemoglobin dissociation curve representing the nonlinear relationship between Po$_2$ and oxygen saturation (Spo$_2$). The curve shifts to the right in response to increased 2,3-BPG concentration within the RBC, severe acidemia, and hypothermia. The dashed line indicates the partial pressure of oxygen at which Hb is 50% saturated under physiologic conditions (P$_{50}$).

process that is reversed by erythrocytic methemoglobin reductase with the subsequent liberation of NO.[6] NO may also bind reversibly with the heme iron of deoxyhemoglobin.[7] In addition, recent evidence suggests that deoxyhemoglobin may have intrinsic nitrite reductase activity, and may generate NO through reduction of nitrite in proportion to its degree of desaturation.[8] These observations point to a role for Hb as an active regulator of microvascular tone through elaboration of NO under conditions of low Po$_2$. At present, there is much interest in the role of Hb in the transport of NO as an endocrine mediator.[9]

MICROVASCULAR DETERMINANTS OF OXYGEN DELIVERY

Adequate levels of both CO and Cao$_2$ are necessary to satisfy the body's oxygen demand, but they are not sufficient. Effective distribution of oxygenated blood throughout the microvascular network (perfusion) is equally important for overall oxygen delivery. A summary of several key concepts linking microvascular structure and function to tissue oxygenation is presented here.

Rheologic Control of Arteriolar Tone

Blood ejected from the left ventricle during systole passes many generations of arterial branching before reaching the arteriolar network. The precapillary arterioles are highly contractile feeder vessels that regulate capillary pressure and the passage of blood into the capillary bed. Arteriolar tone is controlled by a combination of direct autonomic innervation; humoral factors such as catecholamines and vasopressin; and paracrine vasoactive mediators such as NO, endothelin-1, prostacyclin, adenosine-triphosphate (ATP), and endothelium-derived hyperpolarizing factors.[10] Arteriolar vasoconstriction decreases hydrostatic pressure and blood flow within downstream capillaries, and is the major determinant of cardiac afterload.

Local regulation of arteriolar tone involves complex interactions between blood and the vessel wall.[11] Endothelial cells are sensitive transducers of mechanical forces associated with the flow of blood. Fluid shear stresses along the endothelial surface stimulate the release of vasoactive mediators from endothelial cells, most notably the potent vasodilator NO. Arteriolar tone is therefore regulated by changes in blood viscosity and rate of flow, with higher levels of fluid shear leading to enhanced NO production and vasodilation.[6] ATP is also a potent vasodilator that is released from RBCs in response to hypoxia. The efflux of ATP from RBCs has been shown to be proportional to the degree of Hb desaturation, providing a mechanism by which RBCs can respond to low levels of local tissue oxygen tension by triggering vasodilation and increased blood flow to areas of relative hypoxia.[12]

Precapillary Oxygen Delivery

The capillary bed is the site of most nutrient, fluid, and metabolite exchange between the intravascular and interstitial compartments. Historically, the capillary bed has also been considered the primary site of microcirculatory oxygen delivery. This notion originated with the work of the physiologist August Krogh[13,14] in the early twentieth century. Based on observations of the highly regular spatial distribution of capillaries within skeletal muscle, Krogh[13,14] hypothesized that each capillary delivers oxygen to a defined cylindrical volume of surrounding tissue. Together with collaborator Agner Erlang, he developed the first mathematical model of microvascular oxygen delivery (the Krogh-Erlang model), in which the capillary is described as a cylindrical tube with a defined luminal diameter and length. Radial diffusion of oxygen from the central axis of the capillary to the surrounding interstitium was proposed to result in a secondary longitudinal gradient of oxygen, with the highest Po_2 present at the arteriolar end of the capillary, and the lowest Po_2 located at the venous end. The model allowed prediction of the capillary density required to satisfy regional tissue oxygen demand, based on blood oxygen concentration and flow, rate of oxygen consumption by tissue, and capillary diameter.[13,14]

Krogh's[13,14] depiction of the capillary as the primary site of microvascular oxygen delivery remains widely accepted. However, more recent experimental results have highlighted complex and important features of microvascular function that are not accounted for by the Krogh-Erlang model. Based on simultaneous in vivo measurements of Po_2 and oxygen saturation (Spo_2) in small cutaneous arterioles, Duling and Berne[15] described a longitudinal gradient of oxygen within arteriolar segments, indicating that a substantial fraction of oxygen may be delivered to tissues at the precapillary level. Precapillary oxygen delivery has been confirmed in a variety of settings, and in some tissues up to two-thirds of delivered oxygen may exit the microvasculature by diffusion through the walls of small arterioles.[16–18]

The diffusion of oxygen from blood to tissues at the level of the microcirculation is dictated by prevailing gradients of Po_2.[19] As observed by Krogh,[13,14] arterioles and capillaries within skeletal muscle run parallel with myofibers in a highly regular distribution, and this anatomic arrangement leads to predictable longitudinal oxygen gradients within the capillary system. However, in many other tissues, capillary networks have a much less regular organization, and feeder arterioles often exist in close proximity to downstream capillaries or venules. Under these circumstances, complex patterns of oxygen exchange may develop within the microvasculature, in which oxygen diffuses freely among local arterioles, capillaries, and venules in accordance with prevailing gradients.[16,20] This patterns have been confirmed experimentally by the seemingly paradoxic finding of higher oxygen content within blood at the venous end of some capillaries compared with the arterial end.[16] Microvascular arteriovenous oxygen shunting may limit the fraction of overall Do_2 that reaches the capillary bed (**Fig. 3**).

Microvascular Variations in Hematocrit and Blood Viscosity

Blood flow throughout the vascular system is predominantly laminar, in which the cross-sectional area of the moving column of blood shows a parabolic velocity profile,

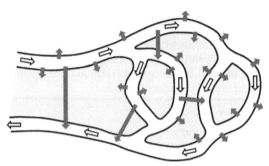

Fig. 3. Patterns of oxygen diffusion in the microcirculation. Open arrows indicate direction of blood flow. Solid arrows indicate hypothetical paths of oxygen diffusion. Oxygen does not solely undergo unidirectional diffusion from the blood to the interstitium, but is exchanged between microvessels in accordance with prevailing gradients of P_{O_2}. (*Adapted from* Ellsworth ML, Ellis CG, Popel AS, et al. Role of microvessels in oxygen supply to tissue. News Physiol Sci 1994;9:122; with permission.)

with the highest flow rates at the center of the moving column, and the lowest flow rates at the luminal surface of the vessel wall. During laminar flow, RBCs undergo axial migration toward the center of the column of flowing blood, resulting in the formation of an approximately 3-μm thick peripheral zone of cell-free plasma (the cell-free layer) adjacent to the endothelial surface.[21] This phase separation has negligible effects on the bulk properties of blood within large vessels, but has profound effects on the properties of blood within arterioles. Within large vessels, blood behaves as a uniform fluid with constant hematocrit (Hct). However, within small arterioles with a luminal diameter of less than 500 μm, blood behaves as a biphasic suspension, the physical properties of which are a function of vessel diameter.

As blood enters progressively smaller vessels, the clustering of RBCs within the central region of the vessel leads to a decrease in the Hct within that vessel, compared with the Hct within the upstream feeder vessel. This reduction in Hct with decreasing vessel diameter was first described by the Swedish physiologist Robin Fahraeus and is referred to as the Fahraeus effect.[22] Essentially, the migration of RBCs into the more rapidly flowing axial portion of the plasma column leads to an increase in the average velocity of RBCs relative to the velocity of overall blood flow. As RBCs pass through a given microvascular segment more quickly, their concentration within that segment decreases proportionally as a necessary condition for conservation of overall RBC flux. The Fahraeus effect is a major determinant of microvascular Hct, especially as vessel diameters approach the size of the transiting RBCs. Although not often taken into account clinically, microvascular Hct is typically less than half of systemic Hct, and under normal conditions can be as low as 10%.[23]

Blood is a complex suspension of deformable cells (mostly RBCs) in a proteinaceous solution (plasma). At the macroscopic level, blood is a non-newtonian fluid with viscoelastic properties. The viscosity of blood is not a fixed property, but varies with Hct, plasma protein concentration, shear rate, and temperature, and is therefore referred to as apparent viscosity.[23] Apparent viscosity is a measure of the resistance of blood to flow, and is an important hemodynamic parameter because increased viscosity requires higher intravascular perfusion pressure, and therefore greater myocardial work for effective circulation. In humans, increased blood viscosity is associated with many forms of cardiovascular disease.[24–26] In animals, pathologic increases in blood viscosity are seen with severe dehydration and hemoconcentration, as well as with polycythemia and some hyperglobulinemias. These conditions lead to obvious perfusion deficits, and are occasionally encountered in surgical patients.

Hct is the primary determinant of the apparent viscosity of blood, and, at given temperature and shear rate, blood viscosity varies exponentially with changes in RBC concentration. Aggregation of RBCs into clusters or rouleaux formations makes a large contribution to blood viscosity; this also underlies its shear dependence, in which increasing flow rate leads to a decrease in viscosity caused by the breakup of RBC aggregates.[27] Given the effect of RBCs on blood viscosity, the Hct reductions that occur within the microvasculature associated with the Fahraeus effect are accompanied by parallel decreases in blood viscosity. This reduction in blood viscosity with decreasing vessel diameter is referred to as the Fahraeus-Lindqvist effect and plays an important role in matching perfusion pressure with microvascular flow.[28]

Plasma Skimming

At microvascular bifurcations, RBCs partition unevenly into daughter branches, with most RBCs entering the branch with the greater volumetric flow. Pouseuille was the first to describe this effect, which is termed plasma skimming.[29] This phenomenon is a direct consequence of the phase separation of flowing blood and formation of the cell-free layer. Its magnitude depends on several factors, including the relative size and geometry of the vascular branches, as well as the velocity of flow and Hct within the parent vessel (**Fig. 4**). Plasma skimming is an important rheologic phenomenon that can lead to significant hemoconcentration within larger daughter branches of successive arterial bifurcations. At the same time, extremely low concentrations of RBCs may develop within smaller daughter vessels. Across successive generations of arteriolar branching, plasma skimming leads to wide regional variations in Hct, viscosity, and flow rate.[30]

ANEMIA

Anemia refers to a decrease in whole-body RBC mass. Quantitative assessment of total RBC mass requires measurement of blood volume; therefore, anemia is most commonly expressed as a subnormal Hb concentration ([Hb]), Hct, or packed cell volume (PCV). PCV is the most commonly used measure of red cell mass in small animal practice. PCV can be used to estimate [Hb] according to the equation $[Hb] \approx PCV/3$. In addition, many automated hematology analyzers report Hct as a calculated value based on the product of the RBC count and the mean corpuscular volume.

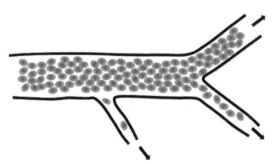

Fig. 4. Plasma skimming at arteriolar bifurcations. Arrows indicate direction of blood flow. Formation of the cell-free layer during laminar flow leads to uneven partitioning of RBCs into daughter branches of microvascular bifurcations and significant regional variations in microvascular Hct.

PCV usually provides a reasonable approximation of total RBC mass; however, animals with acute blood loss can maintain a normal PCV for several hours until plasma volume is restored through fluid shifts or fluid administration. In contrast, aggressive fluid or colloid resuscitation may decrease PCV because of dilutional effects with no change in overall RBC mass. Sequestration or mobilization of RBCs from the spleen may cause acute fluctuations of PCV, with accompanying changes in the oxygen carrying capacity of the blood, despite a constant total RBC mass. These situations are encountered frequently in the perioperative setting; therefore, caution is necessary when interpreting a single PCV in surgical patients. Serial monitoring of PCV is often necessary for accurate assessment of patients' oxygen carrying capacities in the perioperative period.

Anemia is a common condition in surgical patients, and may vary greatly in both severity and chronicity. In animals with intact compensatory responses, anemia is usually well tolerated, and tissue oxygenation can be maintained under resting conditions despite extremely low [Hb].[31] However, the pain, stress, inflammation, and hypermetabolism experienced by animals in the perioperative period may increase global oxygen demand, whereas the effects of anesthetic, analgesic, and sedative agents may simultaneously blunt normal compensatory responses.[32] As a consequence, anemic surgical patients may have an increased Do_2crit and may be uniquely susceptible to tissue hypoxia in the perioperative period (see **Fig. 1**).

PHYSIOLOGIC ADAPTATIONS TO ANEMIA

The overall compensatory physiologic response to anemia consists of an increase in CO and increased o_2ER, along with redistribution of blood flow toward vital organs, particularly the brain and myocardium. These adaptive responses involve variable changes in autonomic tone, alterations in blood viscosity and microvascular flow, and shifts in the oxyhemoglobin dissociation curve.

Cardiac Output

Increased CO is the most consistently documented hemodynamic alteration associated with anemia.[33] Two basic mechanisms underlie the increase in CO during normovolemic anemia: increase in sympathetic stimulation and reduced blood viscosity. In controlled experimental settings, the decreased Cao_2 associated with normovolemic anemia has been shown to increase sympathetic tone through triggering of carotid chemoreceptors,[34] which in turn leads to an increase in CO by direct enhancement of myocardial contractility and heart rate, as well as by augmentation of preload through venoconstriction and mobilization of venous blood.[1] At the same time, anemia causes an intrinsic decrease in blood viscosity that is further compounded by the Fahraeus-Lindqvist effect. The relationship between blood viscosity and CO is complex.[33] The reduction in blood viscosity associated with anemia leads to direct and proportional decreases in cardiac afterload and increases in flow through the microcirculation. Blood viscosity is normally highest in postcapillary venules where increasing Hct and low flow rate facilitate RBC aggregation. Enhanced flow within postcapillary venules inhibits RBC aggregation through increases in local shear and leads to disproportionate reductions in viscosity within venular segments. As a consequence, venous return and cardiac preload are enhanced for a given venous pressure, which further augments CO. In contrast with hypovolemia, in which hemodynamic responses are mediated primarily by the autonomic nervous system, the compensatory increase in CO associated with anemia is attributable mostly to reductions in blood viscosity.[33]

Oxygen Extraction

Anemia also results in an increase in peripheral O_2ER. This increase occurs in all tissues except the myocardium, in which there is high basal O_2ER, and in which any decrease in Do_2 can only be compensated for by coronary vasodilation and increased organ blood flow. With mild to moderate anemia, the CO response is usually sufficient to maintain Do_2 and meet resting tissue oxygen demand; however, as anemia worsens, increased O_2ER becomes an important additional compensatory mechanism. Analogous to the Do_2crit, the threshold value of [Hb] below which compensatory mechanisms become exhausted and global tissue hypoxia develops is the [Hb]crit. In the dog, [Hb]crit corresponds with an Hct of approximately 8%.[35]

O_2ER is enhanced in chronic anemia by shifts in the oxyhemoglobin dissociation curve, which defines the partial pressure of oxygen at which Hb is 50% saturated under physiologic conditions (P_{50}). In the dog, anemia causes a rightward shift in the curve, indicating conditions that favor dissociation of oxygen from Hb, and enhanced peripheral oxygen off-loading. This effect is caused predominantly by increased levels of 2,3-BPG within the erythrocyte, synthesis of which is stimulated by a decrease in intraerythrocytic pH.[36] 2,3-BPG is an allosteric effector that binds to deoxygenated beta-globin subunits and stabilizes the lower oxygen affinity conformation of the Hb tetramer. Upregulation of 2,3-BPG is generally considered to be physiologically advantageous in the context of anemia; however, there is some evidence that Hb with a higher P_{50} (lower oxygen affinity) facilitates the formation of hypoxic foci by off-loading oxygen within oxygenated tissue regions at the expense of less oxygenated regions.[37] 2,3-BPG levels decrease markedly in stored canine blood, which may limit the oxygen carrying capacity of RBCs that are transfused after prolonged periods of storage.[36] Less is known regarding the effect of anemia on the oxyhemoglobin dissociation curve in cats; however, feline erythrocytes contain very little 2-3-BPG.[38] Moreover, feline Hb shows a higher P_{50} and greater cooperativity than that of many other species, indicating a stronger tendency to release oxygen in the periphery.[39,40]

Decreased temperature and acidemia also cause a rightward shift in the oxyhemoglobin dissociation curve; however, the clinical relevance of these effects is debated. In particular, physiologically relevant decreases in pH have very small effects on the P_{50}. The effects of pH on the oxyhemoglobin dissociation curve are thought to be mostly indirect, through stimulation of 2,3-BPG synthesis.[33,41]

CLINICAL APPROACH TO ANEMIC PATIENTS

In-depth discussion of the general clinical and diagnostic approach to anemic patients can be found elsewhere, and readers are referred to several excellent sources.[42–44] In general, clinical signs of anemia are nonspecific, and there is considerable overlap in the physical manifestations of anemia and hypovolemia. One of the cardinal rules of perioperative patient assessment is that hypovolemia must be addressed before the physiologic impacts of anemia can be adequately judged, especially in relation to acute blood loss. Even though blood loss leads to an immediate decrease in the oxygen carrying capacity of the blood, the hemodynamic abnormalities observed in animals with acute hemorrhage are overwhelmingly attributable to hypovolemia and associated perfusion deficits, and not anemia per se.

Assessment of Tissue Oxygenation

In surgical patients, assessment of tissue oxygenation is most commonly based on a combination of physical examination findings, blood gas analysis, oximetry, and plasma lactate measurements. Physical examination findings such as pallor, tachypnea and/or hyperpnea, tachycardia, and aberrant pulse quality can suggest the presence of compensatory responses to anemia, but are generally nonspecific. Arterial blood gas analysis may show a respiratory alkalosis secondary to increased ventilation. However, it is important to remember that normal compensatory hemodynamic and ventilatory responses to anemia may be reduced or absent in anesthetized or sedated patients. Cao_2 is rarely measured clinically, but can be calculated based on Equation 3. Cao_2 is reduced in anemic states, although this does not necessarily indicate inadequate tissue oxygenation unless the reduction is severe. In rare instances in which CO and Cvo_2 measurements are available, o_2ER may be determined. A global o_2ER approaching 50% is generally considered to herald the onset of severe tissue hypoxia[1,35]; however, o_2ER is an insensitive indicator of regional or organ-specific oxygen debt. Pulse oximetry is a commonly used tool for perioperative monitoring of Spo_2; however, anemia does not affect oximetric measurements, thus Spo_2 values remain normal even with severe Hct reduction.

Plasma lactate concentration is a useful and important measure of anaerobic tissue metabolism, and an increased lactate level generally indicates supply-limited Vo_2.[45] Lactate concentration at any given point in time represents a balance between production and metabolism, thus serial lactate measurements are often important. In normovolemic dogs, increased plasma lactate level is a reliable indicator of tissue hypoxia; however, as a global measure, lactate lacks sensitivity for detection of early or regional tissue hypoxia.

These physical, hemodynamic, and biochemical parameters are important clinical variables, but they provide limited information on the adequacy of tissue oxygenation, especially at the regional level. Functional capillary density (FCD) is a parameter of microvascular perfusion that is widely used in microvascular research and that has been shown to correlate well with tissue oxygenation at the microscopic level.[46–48] FCD is defined as the total length of RBC-perfused capillaries within a defined area and is measured by specialized video-microscopic monitoring of capillary beds within small regions of tissue. Capillary pressure and blood viscosity seem to be the primary determinants of FCD.[46] Restoration of FCD is highly correlated with survival following resuscitation from experimental hemorrhagic shock, independently of the oxygen carrying capacity of the blood.[47,49] FCD is an emerging technique for clinical assessment of microvascular perfusion in humans,[50–52] and has also been used in dogs for evaluation of the microhemodynamic effects of fluid administration during ovariohysterectomy.[53]

Methods for Enhancing Oxygen Delivery and Tissue Oxygenation

Under normal conditions, dissolved oxygen accounts for a small fraction of overall Do_2. However, increasing the inspired concentration of oxygen can enhance Do_2 by increasing the amount of dissolved oxygen in the plasma.[54] Per Equation 3, in an animal breathing 100% oxygen with a [Hb] of 6 g/dL and Pao_2 of 450 mm Hg, dissolved oxygen can account for more than 20% of overall Do_2. This effect was shown clearly in a human study of severe normovolemic anemia in which an increase in Pao_2 to 400 mm Hg was associated with hemodynamic improvements equivalent to 3 g/dL of circulating Hb.[55]

Transfusion of RBCs remains a common clinical intervention to improve oxygen carrying capacity in anemic patients, especially in the perioperative setting. In humans, it has been estimated that approximately 50% of all units of transfused RBCs are administered to surgical patients.[56] Perioperative use of RBC transfusions in veterinary practice has not been specifically reported; however, in one large retrospective study, only 5% of transfused units of RBCs were given to surgical patients.[57] Canine and feline blood products along with their storage and use has been reviewed.[58]

RBC transfusion has been reported to improve most measured parameters of oxygen delivery in small animals, and it is generally accepted that the clinical benefits associated with the transfusion of RBCs derive from increased Do_2.[59] However, compelling experimental results suggest that the beneficial effects of transfusion may be attributable largely to improvements in the rheologic properties of blood and normalization of microvascular flow, independent of increases in oxygen carrying capacity of the blood.[60]

Studies using the hamster window chamber system, in which detailed in vivo measurements of microvascular function and tissue oxygenation can be performed on awake animals, have shown that extreme anemia leads to deficits in tissue oxygenation associated with reduced FCD. In this experimental setting, blood transfusion leads to normalization of both FCD and tissue oxygenation.[61] However, in an elegant series of studies, it was shown that both FCD and tissue oxygenation were also restored with transfusion of RBCs in which Hb was converted to methemoglobin, thereby rendering the cells incapable of oxygen transport.[46] Similarly, increasing plasma viscosity by transfusion of a high-molecular-weight alginate-based plasma expander resulted in significant improvements in FCD and tissue oxygenation, with no change in Hct.[62] This increase in microvascular perfusion was associated with increased endothelial production of NO triggered by increased shear stresses imposed on the vascular wall.[62] These studies and others point to reduced blood viscosity as a major contributor to the loss of FCD and defects in tissue oxygenation that occur in severe anemia.[37,49,63,64] The mechanism involves critical decreases in fluid shear with attendant declines in NO production and peripheral vasoconstriction, along with accentuated plasma skimming effects. There is a tight correlation between the level of blood viscosity that leads to loss of FCD and the plasma [Hb] below which Vo_2 becomes supply dependent. This correlation has led to the notion that the conventional transfusion trigger, defined as the Hct below which tissues become at risk for hypoxia, may simultaneously be a viscosity threshold, below which tissues become vulnerable to hypoperfusion because of critical decreases in FCD and microcirculatory collapse.[37]

SUMMARY

Maintenance of adequate oxygen delivery is a critical facet of perioperative care, but clinical assessment of tissue oxygenation remains challenging. Anemia reflects a decreased oxygen carrying capacity of the blood and its significance in the perioperative setting relates largely to the associated risk of insufficient oxygen delivery and cellular hypoxia. From the microcirculatory perspective, oxygen carrying capacity and flow characteristics of blood are closely connected, and the effect of anemia on blood rheology and perfusion should not be disregarded. Meaningful clinical measures of tissue oxygenation are needed in veterinary practice. In the meantime, clinicians must rely on evaluation of a patient's hemodynamic and ventilatory performance, along with biochemical and hemogasometric measurements. Blood transfusion is used commonly for treatment of perioperative anemia, and may improve tissue oxygenation by normalizing the rheologic properties of blood and enhancing perfusion, independent of increases in oxygen carrying capacity.

REFERENCES

1. Chapler CK, Cain SM. The physiologic reserve in oxygen carrying capacity: studies in experimental hemodilution. Can J Physiol Pharmacol 1986;64:7–12.

2. Schechter AN. Hemoglobin research and the origins of molecular medicine. Blood 2008;112:3927–38.
3. Ryter SW, Otterbein LE. Carbon monoxide in biology and medicine. Bioessays 2004;26:270–80.
4. Jensen FB. Red blood cell pH, the Bohr effect, and other oxygenation-linked phenomena in blood O_2 and CO_2 transport. Acta Physiol Scand 2004;182:215–27.
5. Ulker P, Sati L, Celik-Ozenci C, et al. Mechanical stimulation of nitric oxide synthesizing mechanisms in erythrocytes. Biorheology 2009;46:121–32.
6. Singel DJ, Stamler JS. Chemical physiology of blood flow regulation by red blood cells: the role of nitric oxide and S-nitrosohemoglobin. Annu Rev Physiol 2005;67:99–145.
7. Gladwin MT, Ognibene FP, Pannell LK, et al. Relative role of heme nitrosylation and beta-cysteine 93 nitrosation in the transport and metabolism of nitric oxide by hemoglobin in the human circulation. Proc Natl Acad Sci U S A 2000;97:9943–8.
8. Gladwin MT, Schechter AN, Kim-Shapiro DB, et al. The emerging biology of the nitrite anion. Nat Chem Biol 2005;1:308–14.
9. Schechter AN, Gladwin MT. Hemoglobin and the paracrine and endocrine functions of nitric oxide. N Engl J Med 2003;348:1483–5.
10. Segal SS. Regulation of blood flow in the microcirculation. Microcirculation 2005;12:33–45.
11. Baskurt OK, Yalcin O, Meiselman HJ. Hemorheology and vascular control mechanisms. Clin Hemorheol Microcirc 2004;30:169–78.
12. Jagger JE, Bateman RM, Ellsworth ML, et al. Role of erythrocyte in regulating local O_2 delivery mediated by hemoglobin oxygenation. Am J Physiol Heart Circ Physiol 2001;280:H2833–9.
13. Krogh A. The number and distribution of capillaries in muscles with calculations of the oxygen pressure head necessary for supplying the tissue. J Physiol 1919;52:409–15.
14. Krogh A. The supply of oxygen to the tissues and the regulation of the capillary circulation. J Physiol 1919;52:457–74.
15. Duling BR, Berne RM. Longitudinal gradients in periarteriolar oxygen tension. A possible mechanism for the participation of oxygen in local regulation of blood flow. Circ Res 1970;27:669–78.
16. Ellsworth ML, Pittman RN. Arterioles supply oxygen to capillaries by diffusion as well as by convection. Am J Physiol 1990;258:H1240–3.
17. Ivanov KP, Derry AN, Vovenko EP, et al. Direct measurements of oxygen tension at the surface of arterioles, capillaries and venules of the cerebral cortex. Pflugers Arch 1982;393:118–20.
18. Sharan M, Vovenko EP, Vadapalli A, et al. Experimental and theoretical studies of oxygen gradients in rat pial microvessels. J Cereb Blood Flow Metab 2008;28:1597–604.
19. Pittman RN. Oxygen gradients in the microcirculation. Acta Physiol (Oxf) 2011;202:311–22.
20. Ellsworth ML, Ellis CG, Popel AS, et al. Role of microvessels in oxygen supply to tissue. News Physiol Sci 1994;9:119–23.
21. Pries AR, Secomb TW, Gaehtgens P. Biophysical aspects of blood flow in the microvasculature. Cardiovasc Res 1996;32:654–67.
22. Goldsmith HL, Cokelet GR, Gaehtgens P. Robin Fahraeus: evolution of his concepts in cardiovascular physiology. Am J Physiol 1989;257:H1005–15.

23. Lipowsky H. Microrheology of blood flow in the microcirculation. In: Shepro D, editor. Microvascular research: biology and pathology. Burlington (MA): Elsevier; 2005. p. 233–8.
24. Cicco G, Cicco S. The influence of oxygen supply, hemorheology and microcirculation in the heart and vascular systems. Adv Exp Med Biol 2010;662:33–9.
25. Kesmarky G, Kenyeres P, Rabai M, et al. Plasma viscosity: a forgotten variable. Clin Hemorheol Microcirc 2008;39:243–6.
26. Sloop G, Holsworth RE Jr, Weidman JJ, et al. The role of chronic hyperviscosity in vascular disease. Ther Adv Cardiovasc Dis 2015;9:19–25.
27. Baskurt OK, Meiselman HJ. Erythrocyte aggregation: basic aspects and clinical importance. Clin Hemorheol Microcirc 2013;53:23–37.
28. Pries AR, Neuhaus D, Gaehtgens P. Blood viscosity in tube flow: dependence on diameter and hematocrit. Am J Physiol 1992;263:H1770–8.
29. Skalak R, Chien S. Capillary flow: history, experiments and theory. Biorheology 1981;18:307–30.
30. Ellis CG, Jagger J, Sharpe M. The microcirculation as a functional system. Crit Care 2005;9(Suppl 4):S3–8.
31. Champion T, Pereira Neto GB, Camacho AA. Effects of acute normovolemic anemia on hemodynamic parameters and Acid-base balance in dogs. Vet Med Int 2011;2011:829054.
32. Van der Linden P, De Hert S, Mathieu N, et al. Tolerance to acute isovolemic hemodilution. Effect of anesthetic depth. Anesthesiology 2003;99:97–104.
33. Hebert PC, Van der Linden P, Biro G, et al. Physiologic aspects of anemia. Crit Care Clin 2004;20:187–212.
34. Hatcher JD, Chiu LK, Jennings DB. Anemia as a stimulus to aortic and carotid chemoreceptors in the cat. J Appl Physiol Respir Environ Exerc Physiol 1978; 44:696–702.
35. Schwartz S, Frantz RA, Shoemaker WC. Sequential hemodynamic and oxygen transport responses in hypovolemia, anemia, and hypoxia. Am J Physiol 1981; 241:H864–71.
36. Ou D, Mahaffey E, Smith JE. Effect of storage on oxygen dissociation of canine blood. J Am Vet Med Assoc 1975;167:56–8.
37. Tsai AG, Hofmann A, Cabrales P, et al. Perfusion vs. oxygen delivery in transfusion with "fresh" and "old" red blood cells: the experimental evidence. Transfus Apher Sci 2010;43:69–78.
38. Bunn HF. Differences in the interaction of 2,3-diphosphoglycerate with certain mammalian hemoglobins. Science 1971;172:1049–50.
39. Hamilton MN, Edelstein SJ. Cat hemoglobin. pH dependence of cooperativity and ligand binding. J Biol Chem 1974;249:1323–9.
40. Herrmann K, Haskins S. Determination of P_{50} for feline hemoglobin. J Vet Emerg Crit Care (San Antonio) 2005;15:26–31.
41. Hebert J, Hu LQ, Biro G. Review of physiologic mechanisms in response to anemia. Can Med Assoc J 1997;156:S27–39.
42. Ahn AC, Haskin S. Approach to the anemic patient. In: Bonagura JK, Kirk R, editors. Kirk's current veterinary therapy XII. Philadelphia: WB Saunders; 1995. p. 447–51.
43. Rentko V, Clark S. Hematopoietic dysfunction. In: Slatter D, editor. Textbook of small animal surgery. 3rd edition. Philadelphia: Elsevier; 2003. p. 1030–3.
44. Willard M, Tvedten H. Small animal clinical diagnosis by laboratory methods. St. Louis (MO): Elsevier; 2012.
45. Sharkey LC, Wellman ML. Use of lactate in small animal clinical practice. Vet Clin North Am Small Anim Pract 2013;43:1287–97, vi.

46. Cabrales P, Martini J, Intaglietta M, et al. Blood viscosity maintains microvascular conditions during normovolemic anemia independent of blood oxygen-carrying capacity. Am J Physiol Heart Circ Physiol 2006;291:H581–90.

47. Kerger H, Saltzman DJ, Menger MD, et al. Systemic and subcutaneous microvascular Po_2 dissociation during 4-h hemorrhagic shock in conscious hamsters. Am J Physiol 1996;270:H827–36.

48. Tsai AG, Friesenecker B, McCarthy M, et al. Plasma viscosity regulates capillary perfusion during extreme hemodilution in hamster skinfold model. Am J Physiol 1998;275:H2170–80.

49. Cabrales P, Intaglietta M, Tsai AG. Transfusion restores blood viscosity and reinstates microvascular conditions from hemorrhagic shock independent of oxygen carrying capacity. Resuscitation 2007;75:124–34.

50. Bonamy AK, Martin H, Jorneskog G, et al. Lower skin capillary density, normal endothelial function and higher blood pressure in children born preterm. J Intern Med 2007;262:635–42.

51. Genzel-Boroviczeny O, Christ F, Glas V. Blood transfusion increases functional capillary density in the skin of anemic preterm infants. Pediatr Res 2004;56:751–5.

52. Sakr Y, Chierego M, Piagnerelli M, et al. Microvascular response to red blood cell transfusion in patients with severe sepsis. Crit Care Med 2007;35:1639–44.

53. Silverstein DC, Cozzi EM, Hopkins AS, et al. Microcirculatory effects of intravenous fluid administration in anesthetized dogs undergoing elective ovariohysterectomy. Am J Vet Res 2014;75:809–17.

54. Roberson RS, Bennett-Guerrero E. Impact of red blood cell transfusion on global and regional measures of oxygenation. Mt Sinai J Med 2012;79:66–74.

55. Feiner JR, Finlay-Morreale HE, Toy P, et al. High oxygen partial pressure decreases anemia-induced heart rate increase equivalent to transfusion. Anesthesiology 2011;115:492–8.

56. Patel MS, Carson JL. Anemia in the preoperative patient. Med Clin North Am 2009;93:1095–104.

57. Hann L, Brown DC, King LG, et al. Effect of duration of packed red blood cell storage on morbidity and mortality in dogs after transfusion: 3,095 cases (2001–2010). J Vet Intern Med 2014;28:1830–7.

58. Kisielewicz C, Self IA. Canine and feline blood transfusions: controversies and recent advances in administration practices. Vet Anaesth Analg 2014;41:233–42.

59. Kisielewicz C, Self I, Bell R. Assessment of clinical and laboratory variables as a guide to packed red blood cell transfusion of euvolemic anemic dogs. J Vet Intern Med 2014;28:576–82.

60. Tsai AG, Intaglietta M. High viscosity plasma expanders: volume restitution fluids for lowering the transfusion trigger. Biorheology 2001;38:229–37.

61. Cabrales P. Effects of erythrocyte flexibility on microvascular perfusion and oxygenation during acute anemia. Am J Physiol Heart Circ Physiol 2007;293:H1206–15.

62. Tsai AG, Acero C, Nance PR, et al. Elevated plasma viscosity in extreme hemodilution increases perivascular nitric oxide concentration and microvascular perfusion. Am J Physiol Heart Circ Physiol 2005;288:H1730–9.

63. Cabrales P, Tsai AG, Winslow RM, et al. Extreme hemodilution with PEG-hemoglobin vs. PEG-albumin. Am J Physiol Heart Circ Physiol 2005;289:H2392–400.

64. Castro C, Ortiz D, Palmer AF, et al. Hemodynamics and tissue oxygenation after hemodilution with ultrahigh molecular weight polymerized albumin. Minerva Anestesiol 2014;80:537–46.

Oxygenation and Ventilation

 CrossMark

Elizabeth A. Rozanski, DVM

KEYWORDS

- Hypoxemia • Hypoventilation • Mechanical ventilation • Blood gas analysis
- Postoperative

KEY POINTS

- Anticipation of oxygenation and ventilation abnormalities is very helpful in preventing complications.
- Respiratory failure may be due to ventilatory or oxygenation defects.
- Identification of the key abnormalities is essential to treating the patient.
- Intermittent positive pressure ventilation (PPV) may be required to support the patient until recovery and subsequent discharge home.

Perioperative and postoperative care of critically ill animals are vital to a good outcome in patients requiring a surgical procedure. Hypoxemia and/or inadequate ventilation contributes to patient morbidity and mortality if left unsupported. It is ideal to prevent respiratory dysfunction from developing if possible, rather than to play catch-up after failure has occurred.

PREDICTING RESPIRATORY CONCERNS
Evaluation

In a postsurgical intensive care unit (ICU), preparation for a potentially challenging recovery is vital. In smaller hospitals, where all cases are known, it may be easier to keep track of the emerging postoperative case. However, in larger specialty hospitals and academic centers, it may be hard to know all the cases "in motion." The surgical schedule for the day should be carefully perused for cases with known or suspected challenging recoveries. The emergency service clinician should discuss critical admits with planned urgent surgical interventions with the criticalist. If possible, surgeons should be questioned about the extent of the planned intervention, and any preoperative imaging should be reviewed with a radiologist. Critical surgical procedures, when feasible, should go as early in the day as possible to prevent late-day recoveries. For

The author has nothing to disclose.
Section of Critical Care, Cummings School of Veterinary Medicine, Tufts University, 55 Willard Street, North Grafton, MA 01536, USA
E-mail address: Elizabeth.rozanski@tufts.edu

Vet Clin Small Anim 45 (2015) 931–940
http://dx.doi.org/10.1016/j.cvsm.2015.04.001
0195-5616/15/$ – see front matter © 2015 Elsevier Inc. All rights reserved.

vetsmall.theclinics.com

patients with anticipated potential blood loss (eg, adrenalectomy with vena caval invasion), the patient's blood type should be determined and the blood bank resources should be evaluated in case of the potential for massive transfusion. As the surgical procedure is coming to an end, the attending anesthesiologist and receiving criticalist should review the case and discuss postoperative care, including provision of analgesics. The ICU nursing team should be similarly rounded as to the patient's expected arrival time and medical, surgical, and nursing concerns.

Postoperative respiratory complications may be divided into hypoventilation and hypoxemia. Even apparently healthy dogs may desaturate during recovery.[1] However, in healthy animals, oxygenation and ventilation typically return to normal quickly postoperatively. In more seriously ill animals, postoperative prolonged respiratory dysfunction may be loosely divided into difficulty moving air or difficulty with gas exchange. Difficulty moving air includes conditions such as upper airway obstruction, chest wall and diaphragmatic diseases, and severe neuromuscular disease such as cervical intervertebral disk disease (IVDD), while difficulties with gas exchange include conditions such as pneumonia, pulmonary edema, or atelectasis.

TYPES OF SURGICAL PROCEDURES

The following are the surgical procedures that may require significant care from a respiratory perspective postoperatively:

1. Airway: Upper airway surgery in general may be fraught with difficulty recovering from anesthesia because of airway swelling and/or hemorrhage. Breathing against a fixed obstruction can worsen airway edema, which may further narrow the lumen and perpetuate respiratory distress. In addition, transient upper airway obstruction may result in the formation of noncardiogenic pulmonary edema and aspiration of blood or stomach contents and may lead to aspiration pneumonia.
2. Thoracotomy: Exploration of the chest cavity may be performed via a median sternotomy or lateral thoracotomy, depending on the goals of the surgery. Although the choice of the surgical approach is at the discretion of the surgeon, it is important for the managing criticalist to participate in the discussion preoperatively. Open thoracotomy is standard in most small animal practices; however, because current limitations to advancing minimally invasive surgeries are primarily related to equipment and techniques, these will likely be overcome in coming years. As thoracoscopic procedures continue to evolve in animals, it is likely that more and more cases will be performed using minimally invasive techniques. Lung biopsies may also be performed via a keyhole (limited approach), and caudal lung lesions may sometimes be accessed via a transdiaphragmatic approach, which may limit morbidity. Postoperative respiratory dysfunction after thoracic surgery may reflect pain, atelectasis associated with positioning, pleural space disease, pneumonia, vasculitis, or pulmonary embolism. Mild pulmonary hypertension may be associated with a large resection.[2]
3. Abdominal celiotomy: Abdominal surgery ranges from limited approaches to the caudal abdomen such as cystotomy to more extensive procedures such as abdominal sepsis from a gastrointestinal perforation or gastric dilatation volvulus. Respiratory dysfunction after abdominal surgery may be due to a variety of causes, with the most serious being acute respiratory distress syndrome (ARDS) associated with intra-abdominal sepsis and/or aspiration pneumonia.
4. Neurosurgical procedures: The most common procedures include laminectomies and craniotomies. Pulmonary complications associated with neurosurgical procedures include primarily hypoventilation, which is most common in cervical IVDD

and more rarely complications after craniotomies.[3] Ascending myelomalacia, although rare, also results in altered ventilation and ultimately respiratory failure.[4]

5. Brachycephalic animals: A separate category for animals with brachycephalic confirmation undergoing any procedure involving anesthesia is warranted. Anesthetic recovery should always be carefully observed, and anxious patients should not be allowed to pant and whine before the procedure because this can magnify airway swelling and edema.[5] Bulldogs in particular are also prone to gastroesophageal reflux and should be closely monitored for regurgitation and the potential for pneumonia. In the author's hospital, a brachycephalic protocol has been developed and implemented (**Box 1**).

6. Heart failure: Although in most cases is it is preferable to avoid general anesthesia in patients with active heart failure, if it is required for a life-threatening condition or one with severe effect on quality of life, intensive postoperative care should be anticipated. Dogs with mitral regurgitation with preserved contractile function tend to have less difficulty recovering from anesthesia than patients with dilated cardiomyopathies. In all cases, the anesthetic time should be limited and cardiovascularly sparing drugs should be used as much as possible. The clinician should recall that propofol, although short acting, is a profound cardiovascular depressant, and combination protocols with opioids or etomidate may be preferable. Fluid support should be carefully titrated and limited as much as possible.

IMMEDIATE POSTOPERATIVE SUPPORT

The patient should be carefully observed during the recovery period from anesthesia. Supplemental heat should be provided if needed. Supplemental oxygen and suction should be available. Pulse oximetry and capnography may be used to monitor for any apparent pulmonary dysfunction, although limitations exist for both these noninvasive techniques. Using a pulse oximeter, it may be challenging to get an accurate waveform in a patient with darkly pigmented mucous membranes or one with panting or venous distension, which may interfere with the determination of oxygen saturation. Less well recognized, but perhaps more importantly, the end-tidal carbon dioxide ($ETCO_2$) monitor might reflect an acceptable value in millimeters of mercury while the patient is truly hypoventilating; this is because as the patient hypoventilates, the anatomic dead space is maintained. Thus a proportionally higher amount of venous CO_2 returns to the lung and diffuses into the alveolar space; however, when that gas is exhaled, it is diluted with anatomic dead space gas, which contains negligible CO_2, which subsequently results in the appearance of a normal $ETCO_2$. In all cases, if there is any doubt to the efficacy of oxygenation or ventilation, arterial blood gas should be considered.

Specifically, respiratory rate and effort should be closely monitored, as should mucous membrane color, capillary refill time, heart rate, and pulse quality. Any hemorrhage or secretions on the endotracheal tube should be noted and possibly saved for cytology or culture. Thoracic radiography may provide vital clues, but occasionally, atelectasis associated with positioning or anesthesia may make interpretation more challenging. Echocardiography is very useful for assessing volume status and addressing the potential for pulmonary thromboembolism. Provisions for postoperative analgesia should be made, and in patients with questionable pulmonary function, reversible agents and local analgesics should be considered.

HYPOXEMIA

Hypoxemia may develop in patients postoperatively because of excessive sedation and body position[6,7] or more ominously, because of the presence of pulmonary

> **Box 1**
> **An example of a brachycephalic flow chart with guidelines to try to limit postanesthetic complications**
>
> *Description of policy*
>
> This SOP covers any type of surgery (soft tissue, orthopedic, neurosurgery, or ophtho).
>
> All bulldog/brachycephalic sedation/anesthesia is performed by the anesthesia department during regular hours.
>
> Any dog with brachycephalic airway syndrome should have procedures done by experienced personnel, for example, blood drawn, catheter placed, or radiographs taken without anesthesia.
>
> *Preoperative:*
>
> Famotidine 1.0 mg/kg subcutaneously or orally every 12 to 24 hours, or omeprazole 1.0 mg/kg orally every 24 hours
>
> Metoclopramide 0.5 mg/kg subcutaneously every 8 hours
>
> Duration of treatment:
>
> 1. With no history of regurgitation or vomiting: initiate just before surgery, continue postoperatively, based on patient status and judgment of clinician
> 2. With history of regurgitation or vomiting/elective sx: initiate 1 week before surgery, continue postoperatively, based on patient status and judgment of clinician
>
> *If only airway surgery is planned:*
>
> - No opioids administered perioperatively
> - In the operating room, immediately before starting airway surgery, DexSP 0.15 mg/kg administered IV (if no NSAID history)
>
> *Postoperatively for all surgical cases:*
>
> Recovery in ICU, or recovery in anesthesia and moved to ICU when extubated
>
> - Place an IV extension line for aggressive dogs
> - Be prepared for temporary tracheostomy/ventilator support
> - Avoid tracheotomy if possible
> - Consider nasotracheal oxygen
> - Consider sedation (eg, dexdomitor CRI) if required. Consult with attending anesthesiologist
> - Monitor temperature if stridor/stertor present
> - Cough watch
> - Check for nasal discharge
> - Avoid restraint if possible
> - Keep owner informed if complications develop
>
> In certain cases some exceptions may be required based on judgment of the clinician.
> *Abbreviations:* CRI, continuous rate infusion; DexSP, dexamethasone sodium phosphate; IV, intravenous; NSAID, nonsteroidal antiinflammatory drug; SOP, standard operating procedure; sx, surgery.

disease, including aspiration pneumonia, pulmonary thromboembolism, volume overload, or least commonly ARDS. Identification of hypoxemia may be through physical examination confirming labored respiration or based on documentation of hypoxemia with arterial blood gas analysis or pulse oximetry. Treatment of hypoxemia requires both the delivery of supplemental oxygen and a search for the underlying cause.

Supplemental oxygen may be provided via several routes, commonly including supplementation via facemask, nasal oxygen, or oxygen cage. In immediately postoperative patients, reintubation for PPV may be considered as well. Nasal oxygen is particularly easy to place in nonbrachycephalic patients recovering from anesthesia. One caveat is that it is essential to recognize that panting may negate some benefit from nasal oxygen. For example, if a dog is panting, and receiving 3 L/min of supplemental oxygen, with an inspiratory flow rate of 1 L/s, with a 50 ms inspiratory time, the fraction of inspired oxygen (Fio_2) would be 25%, whereas if the same dog on 3 L/min was not panting (eg, inspiratory flow rate of 400 mL/s and inspiratory time 1 second), the Fio_2 would be 31%. Nasotracheal oxygen may also be placed postoperatively. To place nasotracheal oxygen, a nasal catheter is placed routinely but advanced into the trachea under direct visualization. It may be easier to retrieve the catheter from the oropharynx and then to direct it manually down the trachea using hemostats.

Recently, the use of high-flow oxygen therapy (HFOT) has been described in veterinary medicine.[8] HFOT is a nasal oxygen delivery system that delivers humidified and heated oxygen to the patient. The additional warmth and heat improves patient tolerance for higher flow rates, up to 60 L/min, which may be adequate to prevent the need for intubation and mechanical ventilation. While the utility of HFOT is still being established in veterinary patients, early evidence suggests the potential for widespread utility (Christine Guenther DVM, DACVECC, Pittsburgh Veterinary Emergency and Specialty Center, December 2014).

If supplemental oxygen is inadequate to restore normoxemia, or if the patient shows evidence of severe fatigue, then PPV should be considered to permit patient comfort and time to search for an underlying cause.

PPV may be life saving and may be delivered using critical care ventilators, using anesthesia ventilators, or even by hand bagging if needed. Noninvasive PPV with continuous positive airway pressure has been used rarely in animals, primarily because of the degree of sedation required to permit the mask to be tolerated. However, in some animals that are heavily sedated or have altered mentation, the mask may be well tolerated and prevent the need to more invasive ventilation (**Fig. 1**).

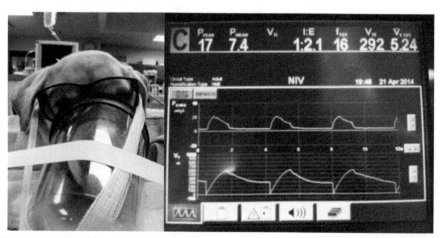

Fig. 1. A dog receiving noninvasive ventilation while recovering from a cervical myleopathy. The glasses are to prevent irritation from the high air flow rate. The ventilator settings are shown on the right.

Most ICUs have dedicated ventilators to support critically ill patients. After electing to begin mechanical ventilation, the clinician needs to set the ventilatory parameters. Some ventilators have built-in algorithms, whereas in older machines, there may be more settings required. In general, the clinician needs to choose the mode of ventilation, the oxygen concentration, the tidal volume, the rate, and the level of positive end-expiratory pressure (PEEP). Volume-limited ventilation means that the ventilator will deliver a set volume, irrespective of the pressure required; this may lead to barotrauma if and when the lung compliance falls. Pressure-limited ventilation means that the tidal volume is limited to a specific inspiratory pressure (eg, 15 cm H_2O); this has the advantage of preventing barotrauma, but if the lungs get less compliant, then hypoventilation (with subsequent hypercarbia) may develop. Ventilation may also be delivered using different modes, the most common being assist/control where the ventilator either delivers breath at a set rate (eg, 15 breaths/min) or senses negative flow at a set rate (Flow trigger); this mode may lead to hyperventilation in dogs that pant. Another major mode is synchronous intermittent mandatory ventilation, which delivers breaths at a preset rate; any additional voluntary efforts by the patient are not supported. There is no mode that does not permit spontaneous efforts. Ventilators may also be used in a spontaneous mode; this mode permits tighter control over the inspired oxygen concentration. PEEP is used to help prevent derecruitment and collapse of the alveoli. It is prudent to recall that the normal negative inspiratory pressure supports cardiac filling, and excessive PEEP in a hemodynamically unstable patient worsens cardiac output. Pressure support is available on some ventilators, and in this mode when a patient initiates the breath, the ventilator completes the breath by supporting to a specific inspiratory pressure (eg, 8 cm H_2O above PEEP).

Almost all dogs and cats require anesthetic depth deep enough to require intubation in order to permit PPV. In dogs and cats with anticipated long-term ventilation, tracheostomy may be considered to reduce the degree of sedation required. There are no ideal sedation/anesthetic agents for ventilation. Pentobarbital was popular for years but is no longer readily available. It should be recalled that propofol is not a particularly safe drug and may be quite cardiovascularly depressing. The ICU at the author's hospital typically uses a combination of continuous rate infusions (CRIs) of opioids (fentanyl), microdoses of alpha-2 agonists, and propofol. Diazepam or midazolam may be added, and ketamine may be useful in some cases. CRI doses that may be useful for ventilated patients include

Fentanyl 2 to 15 µg/kg/h
Ketamine 3 to 10 µg/kg/min
Propofol 0.05 to 0.4 mg/kg/min
Dexmedetomidine load with 1 µg/kg, then 0.5 to 3 µg/kg/h
Lidocaine 50 µg/kg/min (dogs) may be a good addition to some of the other CRIs

The AnaConDa (Sedana Medical AB, Uppsala, Sweden) (http://www.sedanamedical.com/aboutanaconda_or.php) may ultimately prove useful for ventilated patients as well, by allowing the use of anesthetic gases during PPV.

With all patients, the goal is not only to ensure patient comfort and compliance but also to limit excessive anesthesia. However, patients that are undersedated may fight the ventilator and increase work of breathing. Short sedation vacations may be helpful for long-term ventilation. Multimodal approaches may be helpful.

For weaning, transitioning to a propofol CRI may help with more rapid waking. In all cases, long-term infusions may require a longer time frame to metabolize, and over time, alterations in dosing may be required. Seizures have been reported after extended duration of sedation/ventilation. In rare cases, atracurium may be used to prevent bucking the ventilator (eg, patient-ventilator dyssynchrony) but it should be combined with adequate analgesics and long-term use has been associated with prolonged neuromuscular dysfunction after discontinuation of the drug.

In general, the major advantages of PPV are decreasing work of breathing, improving oxygenation, and promoting CO_2 elimination. When considering hypoxemia, a lung-protective approach should be considered, with the idea to limit barotrauma and worsening lung injury. Low tidal volume ventilation is advised in humans, although it has not been explored in dogs with ARDS. One study in beagles confirmed that low tidal volume ventilation is well tolerated in healthy dogs.[9] In humans, ARDSNet has created guidelines for ventilating humans and supports the use of higher PEEP and limiting plateau pressures (www.ARDSNET.gov). Although initially it was believed that the oxygen saturation as measured by pulse oximetry (Spo_2) should be maintained as close to 100% as possible, in humans it has been recognized that an Spo_2 of greater than 88% is adequate and higher values may be associated with perpetuation of lung injury because of barotrauma from the pressures required to result in adequate ventilation.[10]

Major complications of ventilation include progression of the underlying disease. Similar to dialysis in acute kidney injury, ventilation does not specifically treat lung injury, but supports the lung during the time frame required for healing to occur. Pneumothorax is common and should be suspected in the hypoxemic patient treated with higher tidal volumes that acutely desaturate. Ventilator-associated lung injury is possible, and airway colonization (and possibly infection) is another potential complication. Others include "down" patient issues, such as urinary tract infections, peripheral edema including tongue and facial swelling, corneal ulceration, and gastrointestinal ulceration may affect animals being supported with mechanical ventilation.[11]

Weaning from ventilation should be considered when the patient's condition has improved. Practically in veterinary medicine, most ventilator survivors have relatively short clinical courses, although long-term ventilation has been described. Weaning may be attempted if the patient is stable on less than 50% Fio_2, on less than 5 to 6 cm H_2O of PEEP, and importantly with relatively low peak inspiratory pressure (PIP) (eg, <15 cm H_2O or so). If a high PIP is required to maintain adequate oxygenation, then spontaneous ventilation is inadequate and the patient quickly tires and fails weaning.

A search for the underlying cause of hypoxemia is warranted in patients without a clear explanation. Thoracic radiographs may be misleading in the immediate postoperative period but may provide useful clues as to the cause of the pathology if abnormal findings are present. In patients recovering from a thoracotomy, the chest drain should be checked for the presence of air or fluid, and if respiratory distress persists, a diagnostic thoracocentesis may be considered or the thoracic cavity evaluated by thoracic-focused abdominal sonography in trauma (T-FAST) for evidence of fluid, loss, or glide (consistent with pneumothorax). In animals with thoracic or high lumbar spinal fractures, it is not uncommon to have an inadvertent pneumothorax after surgical repair, so this should also be considered in patients with unexplained tachypnea. Echocardiography is exceedingly useful to assess a patient for volume overload and pulmonary thromboembolism and to evaluate cardiac function, and it has the advantage of being able to be performed cage or run-side.[12]

HYPOVENTILATION

Ventilatory failure is defined as a raised $ETCO_2$, with values of greater than 50 mm Hg in an arterial blood gas. In cases in which an arterial blood gas cannot be obtained, a normal pulse oximetry reading while breathing room air effectively excludes hypoventilation.[13] However, if a patient is provided with supplemental oxygen, a normal pulse oximetry reading is not able to guarantee normal CO_2. It should be recalled that in mammals, arterial CO_2 is the primary stimulant for ventilation; however, hypoxemia will also stimulate ventilation. **Table 1** shows changes in arterial blood gas after a Doberman pinscher that was hypoventilating was inadvertently provided supplemental oxygen. Ventilatory failure may develop because of either inadequate ventilatory drive or severe parenchymal disease that limits tidal volume owing to loss of pulmonary compliance. Inadequate ventilatory drive typically occurs after postoperative cervical IVDD or other cervical fracture repairs, or less commonly after craniotomy, chest wall surgery, or resuscitation after cardiopulmonary arrest. In this case, the patient has near-normal lungs but has lost the drive to ventilate or the ability to adequately ventilate. Arterial carbon dioxide concentrations are by definition raised, and at values of greater that 70 mm Hg or so, the accompanying respiratory acidosis further depresses the patient's ventilatory efforts. Severely affected patients require mechanical ventilation, typically with endotracheal tube placement. In patients requiring longer-term support, a tracheostomy may be considered.

Mechanical ventilation of dogs and cats with ventilatory failure may use any mode. For animals that have ineffective but present ventilatory effort, pressure support ventilation, where each patient-initiated breath is supported to a certain level (eg, 6 cm H_2O) above PEEP, may be used, and as ventilatory function returns, the degree of ventilatory support may be decreased until the patient is spontaneously breathing with additional support. In apneic patients, any ventilatory mode may be used to maintain adequate oxygenation and ventilation. In general, in patients with hypoventilation only, limited additional oxygen support should be required, meaning either ventilation using room air or 25% inspired oxygen should be more than adequate. In patients with unexpected apnea, or progressive decrease in ventilatory function, consideration should be given regarding whether any imaging (eg, cervical MRI scan) should be urgently pursued to evaluate for any necessary surgical interventions.

Intravenous respiratory stimulants have been used in infants with apnea of prematurity and occasionally in adults. Beneficial effects are seen from aminophylline, doxapram, and caffeine. Stimulants (eg, caffeine) are occasionally used in neonatal foals, and doxapram is occasionally provided sublingually to neonatal puppies and kittens, although controlled studies about the efficacy of these interventions have not been performed. In anesthetized neonatal foals with respiratory acidosis, doxapram was more effective at restoring ventilation than caffeine.[14]

Table 1
Arterial blood gases, pulse oximetry, and capnography (face mask) from a Doberman pinscher with severe cervical IVDD

Parameters (Units)	At Presentation	After Oxygen Supplementation
pH	7.237	7.021
Pco_2 (mm Hg)	51.3	91.5
Po_2 (mm Hg)	59.7	421.9
HCO_3 (mmol/L)	22	26
Pulse oximetry (%)	93	100
$ETCO_2$ (mm Hg)	47	32

Note the effect of supplemental oxygen on the Pco_2 as well as the inaccuracy in assessing arterial CO_2 by capnography in this hypoventilating dog.

Combined Ventilatory and Oxygenation Failure

Combined failure, with both CO_2 retention and hypoxemia, develops for 2 reasons. The first is when pulmonary parenchymal disease results in such severely decreased compliance that the patient is unable to maintain an effort to effectively exchange gases. For example, in order to generate a tidal volume of 400 mL, normally an inspiratory pressure of 4 cm H_2O would be required, with a resulting compliance of approximately 100 mL/cm H_2O; however, if compliance is reduced by 75% to 25 mL/cm H_2O, an inspiratory pressure of approximately 16 cm H_2O would be required to generate the same 400 mL tidal volume. The work of breathing required to generate 16 cm H_2O inspiratory pressure is tiring, and respiratory fatigue may develop. The patient then decreases his effort to perhaps 8 cm H_2O, and subsequently only 200 mL tidal volume is obtained. The patient may compensate for this for a short time by increasing the respiratory rate, which will maintain a relatively normal minute ventilation. However, in severe cases, pulmonary failure develops. In animals with pulmonary parenchymal disease resulting in increased work of breathing as the cause of hypoventilation, PPV can eliminate the work of breathing and return arterial CO_2 levels to near-normal ranges.

Carbon dioxide retention may also develop in association with severe disease at the alveoli-capillary interface. CO_2 is intrinsically very diffusible, and thus limitations with diffusion are consistent with extreme pulmonary dysfunction. Diffusion impairment will not improve with simple mechanical ventilation. In humans, extracorporeal techniques are being used with increasing frequency to remove CO_2 in conjunction with low tidal volumes to limit perpetuation of lung injury.[15]

SUMMARY

Perioperative and postoperative respiratory support is essential for a good outcome for surgical patients. Adequate oxygenation and ventilation are essential for recovery. Early detection and prompt correction of abnormalities will likely improve outcome (**Box 2**).

Box 2
Guidelines for perioperative and postoperative care of critically ill dogs and cats

1. Early broad-spectrum antibiotic therapy is warranted with any suspicion of pneumonia. While a culture is ideal, untreated pneumonia may be promptly fatal. In large referral hospitals, MDR strains may predominate, and coverage for anticipated pathogens is warranted. Animals receiving antibiotics in the past month are more likely to have MDR infections.

2. Echocardiography is very useful in determining volume status/volume overload, as well as systolic function. Pulmonary hypertension is more common than potentially appreciated.

3. Pulmonary thromboembolism may be a player in some postoperative canine respiratory distress; diagnosis is challenging. The D-dimer is less helpful than anticipated.[16] Echocardiography is often helpful, while CT angiography is considered the gold standard, but requires anesthesia and CT scanner.

4. ARDS is an uncommon but possible cause of postoperative respiratory distress in hospitalized dogs with underlying critical illness. ARDS is a secondary lesion, not a primary disease.

5. Steroids are beneficial in some lung diseases and upper airway fixed and dynamic obstructions, including decompensated tracheal collapse.

Abbreviations: CT, computed tomography; MDR, multidrug resistance.

REFERENCES

1. Campbell VL, Drobatz KJ, Perkowski SZ. Postoperative hypoxemia and hypercarbia in healthy dogs undergoing routine ovariohysterectomy or castration and receiving butorphanol or hydromorphone for analgesia. J Am Vet Med Assoc 2003;222(3):330–6.
2. Anagnostou TL, Pavlidou K, Savvas I, et al. Anesthesia and perioperative management of a pneumonectomized dog. J Am Anim Hosp Assoc 2012;48(2): 145–9.
3. Beal MW, Paglia DT, Griffin GM, et al. Ventilatory failure, ventilator management, and outcome in dogs with cervical spinal disorders: 14 cases (1991-1999). J Am Vet Med Assoc 2001;218(10):1598–602.
4. Okada M, Kitagawa M, Ito D, et al. Magnetic resonance imaging features and clinical signs associated with presumptive and confirmed progressive myelomalacia in dogs: 12 cases (1997-2008). J Am Vet Med Assoc 2010;237(10):1160–5.
5. Hoareau GL, Mellema MS, Silverstein DC. Indication, management, and outcome of brachycephalic dogs requiring mechanical ventilation. J Vet Emerg Crit Care (San Antonio) 2011;21(3):226–35.
6. Rozanski EA, Bedenice D, Lofgren J, et al. The effect of body position, sedation, and thoracic bandaging on functional residual capacity in healthy deep-chested dogs. Can J Vet Res 2010;74(1):34–9.
7. McMillan MW, Whitaker KR, Hughes D, et al. Effect of body position on the arterial partial pressures of oxygen and carbon dioxide in spontaneously breathing, conscious dogs in an intensive care unit. J Vet Emerg Crit Care (San Antonio) 2009;19:564–70.
8. Keir I, Daly J, Haggerty J, et al. High flow oxygen therapy improves PaO2 in dogs with hypoxemia failing traditional oxygen therapy. Proceedings from the 32nd Symposium of the Veterinary Comparative Respiratory Society, Kennett Square (PA): PennVET; 2014.
9. Oura T, Rozanski EA, Buckley G, et al. Low tidal volume ventilation in healthy dogs. J Vet Emerg Crit Care (San Antonio) 2012;22(3):368–71.
10. Hess DR. Ventilatory strategies in severe acute respiratory failure. Semin Respir Crit Care Med 2014;35(4):418–30.
11. Hopper K, Haskins SC, Kass PH, et al. Indications, management, and outcome of long-term positive-pressure ventilation in dogs and cats: 148 cases (1990-2001). J Am Vet Med Assoc 2007;230(1):64–75.
12. DeFrancesco TC. Management of cardiac emergencies in small animals. Vet Clin North Am Small Anim Pract 2013;43(4):817–42.
13. Fu ES, Downs JB, Schweiger JW, et al. Supplemental oxygen impairs detection of hypoventilation by pulse oximetry. Chest 2004;126(5):1552–8.
14. Giguère S, Sanchez LC, Shih A, et al. Comparison of the effects of caffeine and doxapram on respiratory and cardiovascular function in foals with induced respiratory acidosis. Am J Vet Res 2007;68(12):1407–16.
15. Bein T, Weber-Carstens S, Goldmann A, et al. Lower tidal volume strategy (≈ 3 ml/kg) combined with extracorporeal CO2 removal versus 'conventional' protective ventilation (6 ml/kg) in severe ARDS: the prospective randomized Xtravent-study. Intensive Care Med 2013;39(5):847–56.
16. Epstein SE, Hopper K, Mellema MS, et al. Diagnostic utility of D-dimer concentrations in dogs with pulmonary embolism. J Vet Intern Med 2013;27(6):1646–9.

Perioperative Acid-Base and Electrolyte Disturbances

Kari Santoro Beer, DVM, Lori S. Waddell, DVM*

KEYWORDS

- Acidosis • Alkalosis • Electrolytes • Oxygenation • Ventilation

KEY POINTS

- Acid-base and electrolyte abnormalities are common in perioperative patients, and appropriate recognition and treatment is essential to optimize outcome.
- Fluid therapy provides treatment of most metabolic acid-base disturbances.
- Respiratory support, including supplemental oxygen and occasionally mechanical ventilation, may be necessary to correct respiratory disturbances.
- Electrolyte disturbances may be corrected by fluid therapy or a variety of pharmacologic agents.
- Correction of these disorders preoperatively and intraoperatively results in a more stable anesthetic candidate.

INTRODUCTION

Obtaining and interpreting values for blood gases and electrolytes is essential in the management of many perioperative veterinary patients. Metabolic and electrolyte alterations are common in critically ill surgical patients, and can lead to alterations in cardiovascular function, neurologic status, respiratory function, and even response to various drug therapies. Several common preoperative and postoperative conditions are discussed in this article. **Box 1** contains a 6 step method for the interpretation of blood gases, a skill that is needed to diagnose some of the derangements that are discussed in this article. Normal arterial and venous blood gas values for dogs and cats are listed in **Table 1**, and the expected compensatory changes are listed in **Table 2**.

Disclosure: The authors have nothing to disclose.
Intensive Care Unit, Department of Clinical Studies, Matthew J. Ryan Veterinary Hospital, University of Pennsylvania, School of Veterinary Medicine, 3900 Spruce Street, Philadelphia, PA 19104, USA
* Corresponding author.
E-mail address: loriwadd@vet.upenn.edu

Vet Clin Small Anim 45 (2015) 941–952
http://dx.doi.org/10.1016/j.cvsm.2015.04.003

Box 1
Interpreting blood gas results

There are 6 steps required to interpret blood gas results:

1. Determine whether sample is venous or arterial. Either sample type can be used to evaluate overall acid-base status, with the exception of severe shock and postarrest situations, which may result in large discrepancies between arterial and venous samples. Poor tissue perfusion can result in sizable increases in CO_2 and secondary decreases in pH on the venous side despite low to normal CO_2 on the arterial side.

   Although information can be gained about ventilation from a venous sample, only an arterial sample can assess oxygenation.

   If unable to obtain an arterial sample, use pulse oximetry to measure oxygen saturation and a venous sample to evaluate acid-base status and estimate ventilation.

   If the patient is intubated, end-tidal CO_2 can also be used to estimate ventilation, but, with severe pulmonary disease, end-tidal CO_2 can be much lower than $Paco_2$.

2. Assess the patient for acidemia (pH <7.35) or alkalemia (pH >7.45).

   If pH is within normal limits, the patient's body may have compensated for an underlying disturbance or a mixed disturbance may be present. See steps 3 and 4 to evaluate whether metabolic or respiratory disturbances are present despite normal pH.

3. Assess for acidosis.

   Respiratory acidosis is present if $Paco_2$ is greater than 45 mm Hg.

   Metabolic acidosis is present if base excess (BE) is less than −4 mmol/L (or HCO_3^- <19 mmol/L).

4. Assess for alkalosis.

   Respiratory alkalosis is present if $Paco_2$ is less than 35 mm Hg.

   Metabolic alkalosis is present if BE >2 mmol/L (or HCO_3^- >25 mmol/L).

5. Assess oxygenation.

   Normal Pao_2 is 90 to 100 mm Hg. If the patient is on supplemental oxygen, Pao_2 should equal approximately 5 times the fraction of inspired oxygen (Fio_2); the Fio_2 of room air is 21%.

   These rules apply to the normal values listed in **Table 1** for dogs. For cats, substitute the reported normal values for $Paco_2$ and BE from **Table 1** into steps 3 and 4.

6. Determine whether compensatory changes have occurred.

   For example, if a primary metabolic acidosis is present, a compensatory respiratory alkalosis may also exist. Remember the rules of compensation:

   A change in the respiratory or metabolic component of the acid-base status normally induces an opposite compensatory response in an effort to normalize the pH.

   The lungs can compensate quickly by adjusting minute ventilation in a matter of minutes.

   The kidneys compensate more slowly, with compensation beginning within a few hours and maximum compensation taking 4 to 5 days.

   The absence or presence and degree of compensation provide some information about the chronicity of the disturbance (see **Table 2**).

   Overcompensation does not occur.

Table 1
Normal values for canine and feline arterial and venous blood gases

	Arterial Values	Venous Values
Dogs[1]		
pH	7.395 ± 0.03	7.352 ± 0.02
Po_2 (mm Hg)	102.1 ± 6.8	55 ± 9.6
Pco_2 (mm Hg)	36 ± 2.7	42.1 ± 4.4
HCO_3^- (mmol/L)	21.4 ± 1.6	22.1 ± 2
BE (mmol/L)	-1.8 ± 1.6	-2.1 ± 1.7
Cats[2]		
pH	7.34 ± 0.1	7.30 ± 0.08
Po_2 (mm Hg)	102.9 ± 15	38.6 ± 11
Pco_2 (mm Hg)	33.6 ± 7	41.8 ± 9
HCO_3^- (mmol/L)	17.5 ± 3	19.4 ± 4
BE (mmol/L)	-6.4 ± 5	-5.7 ± 5

Abbreviation: BE, base excess.

PREOPERATIVE DERANGEMENTS

Preoperative patients, especially those undergoing emergency procedures, commonly have several acid-base and electrolyte derangements secondary to hypovolemia and underlying systemic illness. The most common abnormalities are discussed here.

Metabolic Acidosis

Metabolic acidosis occurs when endogenous or exogenous acids exceed the body's buffering capacity, resulting in a decrease in pH to less than 7.35. Systemic acidosis is important to recognize and treat because prolonged acidosis results in denaturation of proteins within the body, leading to impaired cellular function; organ dysfunction, including decreased myocardial contractility, ventricular arrhythmias, and fibrillation;

Table 2
Expected compensatory responses

Disorder	Changes	Compensatory Response
Metabolic acidosis	$\downarrow HCO_3^-$	0.7 mm Hg decrease in $Paco_2$ for each 1 mEq/L decrease in HCO_3^-
Metabolic alkalosis	$\uparrow HCO_3^-$	0.7 mm Hg increase in $Paco_2$ for each 1 mEq/L increase in HCO_3^-
Acute respiratory acidosis	$\uparrow Paco_2$	1.5 mEq/L increase in HCO_3^- for each 10 mm Hg increase in $Paco_2$
Chronic respiratory acidosis	$\uparrow Paco_2$	3.5 mEq/L increase in HCO_3^- for each 10 mm Hg increase in $Paco_2$
Acute respiratory alkalosis	$\downarrow Paco_2$	2.5 mEq/L decrease in HCO_3^- for each 10 mm Hg decrease in $Paco_2$
Chronic respiratory alkalosis	$\downarrow Paco_2$	5.5 mEq/L decrease in HCO_3^- for each 10 mm Hg decrease in $Paco_2$

Data from DiBartola SP. Introduction to acid–base disorders. In: DiBartola SP, editor. Fluid, electrolyte, and acid–base disorders in small animal practice, 4th ed. St. Louis: Elsevier Saunders; 2012. p. 231–52.

vasodilation with decreased response to catecholamines; insulin resistance; increased work of breathing (to compensate for a metabolic acidosis); and potentially death. The major causes of metabolic acidosis include lactic acidosis, exogenous acids, ketoacidosis, uremia, and loss of bicarbonate.

Lactic Acidosis

The most common cause of metabolic acidosis is lactate accumulation. Lactate is the end product of anaerobic metabolism; lactic acidosis occurs when plasma lactate is increased in conjunction with a decrease in systemic blood pH.[3,4] Lactic acidosis is common in patients with hypoperfusion or hypoxia, and has also been reported in association with other conditions (sepsis, neoplasia, drugs/toxins, mitochondrial dysfunction, inborn errors of metabolism).[5,6] In addition, an increased lactate level can be seen with end-stage liver failure (because it normally metabolizes most of the lactate produced) or with a focal area of tissue ischemia or necrosis (eg, a loop of infarcted bowel). Two types of lactic acidosis exist: type A and type B. Type A lactic acidosis is more common and occurs with tissue hypoxia and increased lactate production caused by anaerobic glycolysis. Type B lactic acidosis occurs when oxygen delivery is adequate but use of oxygen is impaired, as with altered mitochondrial function or carbohydrate metabolism. There are 3 subtypes of B lactic acidosis: B1 includes diseases that cause decreased lactate clearance, B2 includes drugs or toxins that interfere with oxidative phosphorylation, and B3 includes mitochondrial defects.[7] Although type A lactic acidosis is the likely cause of metabolic acidosis in many perioperative patients, both types likely exist concurrently in many patients, especially those with sepsis.[3,7,8] Diagnosis of lactic acidosis is made by measuring serum L-lactate concentration. Two forms of lactate exist: L-lactate is the most commonly measured and is produced by cellular metabolism in healthy monogastric animals; D-lactate is produced during bacterial glucose metabolism or alternate metabolic pathways in some intoxications or diseases.[8] L-Lactate can be quickly measured on many of the newer blood gas analyzers or with a hand-held point-of-care lactate analyzer. Several factors, including stress, seizures, recent exercise, excitement, food intake, and prolonged venous stasis during collection, can potentially increase lactate concentrations from 2.5 to 10 mmol/L.[3,9] In cats, one study showed a 10-fold increase in lactate levels in healthy cats that were stressed before sample collection, although a more recent study showed no statistical differences in lactate levels with struggling during sampling.[10,11] If measurement of plasma lactate is not possible, it can be suspected when a metabolic acidosis is present on blood gas analysis that is not secondary to diabetic ketoacidosis, renal failure, renal tubular acidosis, or exogenous acids such as ethylene glycol.

In human patients, lactate monitoring is commonly used to guide resuscitation and for prognostication purposes, and numerous studies have shown that as blood lactate concentrations increase, probability of survival decreases.[12–15] More recently in human medicine, emphasis has been placed on monitoring serial lactate concentrations, because studies have shown that patients who clear increased lactate levels have improved outcomes compared with those who do not.[15–18] Several veterinary studies, mostly in dogs, have also shown that lactate can be used to identify hypoperfusion and assess response to therapy.[5,19–24] A notable area of lactate research in canine patients has focused on lactic acidosis with gastric dilatation-volvulus, which can develop secondary to either regional or systemic hypoperfusion.[21,24] Studies have shown correlations between initial plasma lactate concentrations and the presence of gastric necrosis as well as outcome, and more recent studies have shown correlations between lactate clearance and resuscitation and survival.[19–21,24]

Many surgical patients present with a lactic acidosis secondary to hypovolemia, whether they are patients with trauma; acute abdomens, including gastric dilatation-volvulus; septic peritonitis; hemoabdomen, or other causes. Treatment of lactic acidosis is designed to improving oxygen delivery to the tissues. Most commonly, this is corrected by volume resuscitation (assessment of perfusion and fluid balance is discussed by Boller elsewhere in this issue), but, in some cases, providing supplemental oxygen or a hemoglobin source such as packed red blood cells is necessary. Although aggressive fluid therapy may be warranted in some hypovolemic patients, caution should be exercised, especially in septic surgical patients, because recent human studies have shown worse outcomes in septic patients with fluid overload.[25] Bicarbonate administration should never be necessary when a metabolic acidosis is caused by lactate. Without treatment, severe acidosis can lead to vasodilation and hypotension, arrhythmias, decreased cardiac contractility, increased respiratory effort, mental dullness, insulin resistance, and death.[7,8]

Uremia can also result in a severe metabolic acidosis. This condition can be a concern in patients with uroabdomen, ureteral obstructions, or urethral obstruction that cannot be relieved and requires anesthesia and surgery. Treatment consists of appropriate fluid therapy; treatment of concurrent hyperkalemia, if present; as well as sodium bicarbonate therapy, if indicated. In cases of oliguric or anuric acute kidney injury, advanced modalities such as peritoneal dialysis, intermittent hemodialysis, or continuous renal replacement therapy may be recommended.

Hyperkalemia

Severe hyperkalemia can quickly become a life-threatening emergency because of its effects on the cardiovascular system. High potassium levels decrease the transmembrane potassium gradient and depolarize the cell membrane, impairing excitation and conduction. These changes can result in cardiac effects, including bradycardia, atrial standstill, and cardiac arrest. Typical electrocardiogram (ECG) changes include a peaked, narrow T wave (serum potassium concentration >5.5 mEq/L); prolonged QRS complex and PR interval; depressed R wave amplitude and ST segment (>6.5 mEq/L); depressed P wave amplitude (>7 mEq/L); atrial standstill or sinoventricular rhythm (>8.5 mEq/L); and biphasic QRS complexes, ventricular flutter, ventricular fibrillation, or asystole (>10 mEq/L).[26,27] Although experimental studies of hyperkalemia have been shown to induce these specific electrocardiographic changes, the same levels of hyperkalemia may not show parallels in clinical patients, and potassium should always be measured in clinical patients.[27] Patients with just a moderate hyperkalemia may be more at risk for anesthetic complications even if they have not been clinical before anesthesia.[28] In addition, systemic effects, including weakness, flaccid paralysis, respiratory failure, gastrointestinal hypomotility, and hyporeflexia can occur.

Causes of hyperkalemia include decreased excretion of potassium caused by urethral obstruction, rupture of the urinary tract, acute renal failure, hypoadrenocorticism, severe metabolic acidosis, and crush injury. However, many of these causes are surgical, and stabilization of the patient, including normalization of potassium concentration, is necessary before anesthesia and surgery are advisable. Treatment may include intravenous (IV) fluid therapy if the patient is hypovolemic or dehydrated, calcium gluconate, insulin and dextrose, and sodium bicarbonate administration.

Treatment of hyperkalemia involves 3 phases: immediate cardioprotection from life-threatening hyperkalemia, redistribution of serum potassium, and excretion of potassium from the body. Immediate cardioprotection can be achieved with IV calcium gluconate while monitoring the ECG. Calcium gluconate does not decrease the serum K^+ concentration, but does decrease the threshold potential for the cardiac cells, reestablishing the normal difference between resting and threshold potentials. This process helps to normalize membrane excitability within minutes of administration. In dogs and cats, the recommended dose of 10% calcium gluconate is 50 to 150 mg/kg as a slow (5–10 minutes) IV bolus. Administering calcium gluconate too quickly can result in worsening bradycardia and severe ventricular arrhythmias, so an ECG should be monitored while administering. The onset of action is rapid (within 5 minutes) but short acting, so additional steps must be taken to reduce serum potassium levels. Redistribution of serum potassium can be achieved with dextrose and/or regular insulin. Dextrose can be given as an IV bolus (0.5 g/kg) to promote endogenous insulin release and movement of potassium intracellularly, as it is cotransported with glucose. Regular crystalline insulin can be given at the same time at a dose of 0.25 to 0.5 U/kg IV. Exogenous insulin may have a quicker onset of action and a more dramatic reduction in potassium concentration, but hypoglycemia can result. When using insulin and dextrose, it is imperative that dextrose be supplemented in the fluids at 2.5% to 5% in addition to giving a dextrose bolus at the dose mentioned earlier to prevent secondary hypoglycemia. Sodium bicarbonate can also be used to treat hyperkalemia. It promotes movement of potassium intracellularly as hydrogen ions move extracellularly to buffer the bicarbonate. This treatment may be especially helpful in cases with hyperkalemia and a concurrent metabolic acidosis. An IV dose of 1 to 2 mEq/kg of sodium bicarbonate is given slowly over 15 minutes, or the base excess (BE) can be used to calculate the base deficit (base deficit = 0.3 × BE × weight in kilograms) and one-quarter to one-third of that calculated value is given intravenously. Terbutaline can also be used to stimulate Na^+/K^+-ATPase to cause translocation of potassium into the cell.[29] It can be given as a dose of 0.01 mg/kg subcutaneously or intravenously.

The underlying cause of hyperkalemia should be addressed as soon as possible. Preoperatively, this may include relieving a urethral obstruction, providing a method of drainage for a uroabdomen, or improving renal perfusion and increasing urine output in patients with oliguric or anuric acute kidney injury. Although 0.9% NaCl is the hypothetical fluid of choice for hyperkalemia because it contains no additional potassium, administration of any balanced electrolyte solution (Normosol-R, Plasmalyte-A, or lactated Ringer solution [LRS]) helps to dilute the serum potassium concentration. One study in cats with urethral obstruction comparing the use of 0.9% NaCl and Normosol-R showed that the use of a balanced electrolyte solution such as Normosol-R may allow more rapid normalization of acid-base abnormalities and does not affect the rate of normalization of serum potassium.[30]

Once the patient's potassium has been stabilized, anesthesia and surgery to correct the underlying problem can be considered. During anesthesia, the patient's ventilation should be monitored carefully because hypercapnia may decrease pH and result in release of potassium from cells.[28] In severe cases, the treatments mentioned earlier may not be sufficient treatment of the hyperkalemia. In these cases, peritoneal dialysis or, ideally, hemodialysis is indicated. If surgery is attempted in patients with hyperkalemia that has not/cannot be corrected medically, it should be kept in mind that these cases are poor anesthetic candidates and are at high risk of cardiac arrest. Every attempt should be made to stabilize the potassium and its cardiovascular effects before anesthesia.

Hypochloremic Metabolic Alkalosis

This preoperative derangement is classically seen with high gastrointestinal obstruction, although a recent study reported that hypochloremic, hypokalemic metabolic alkalosis is seen with proximal and distal foreign body obstructions in dogs.[31] Other causes of metabolic alkalosis identified in dogs and cats in a recent retrospective study include respiratory disease, furosemide administration, and renal disease.[32] With a gastrointestinal obstruction, vomiting results in a loss of hydrogen, sodium, potassium, chloride, and water, resulting in extracellular fluid and intravascular volume depletion, and development of a hypochloremic metabolic alkalosis. Gastric fluid has a very high concentration of chloride (150 mEq/L). Continued loss of hydrogen in the vomitus creates a metabolic alkalosis, because 1 bicarbonate molecule is produced for every hydrogen ion. The concurrent volume depletion stimulates the kidneys to reabsorb sodium. Because of continued loss of hydrogen and chloride and lack of intake of dietary salt, a deficit of chloride occurs. These patients are in a volume-depleted state that activates the renin angiotensin system. As the kidneys reabsorb sodium, they are unable to reabsorb chloride because of chloride depletion. Instead, they rely on reabsorption of sodium in place of potassium and hydrogen. This process results in hypokalemia and a paradoxic aciduria.[1]

Treatment should be designed to correct the underlying cause after correcting intravascular volume and chloride concentrations. The fluid therapy of choice for volume replacement is 0.9% NaCl because of its high chloride concentration. Potassium should be supplemented, if indicated, once any boluses have been completed. The metabolic alkalosis may take several days to resolve, even with appropriate fluid therapy. Once the patient has been stabilized cardiovascularly, the underlying cause can be addressed. Surgery for removal of a pyloric foreign body or for treatment of pyloric hypertrophy is often indicated. Care should be taken while the animal is under anesthesia to avoid hyperventilation. A compensatory respiratory acidosis will be present because of the metabolic alkalosis, and hyperventilation abolishes this compensatory response and results in severe alkalemia.[1]

INTRAOPERATIVE DERANGEMENTS
Hypoxemia/Hypercapnia

Hypoxemia is defined as a partial pressure of oxygen (Pa_{O_2}) less than 80 mm Hg or arterial hemoglobin saturation less than 95%. The 3 major causes of hypoxemia are low inspired oxygen, hypoventilation, and venous admixture.[33] In the perioperative period, hypoxemia commonly occurs secondary to all of these causes. Low inspired oxygen can occur with anesthetic equipment complications (eg, neglecting to turn on an oxygen source or running out of oxygen from a tank). Hypoventilation is defined as an increased Pa_{CO_2} (usually >45 mm Hg) and can rapidly cause a life-threatening respiratory acidosis. Causes can include impairment of the normal respiratory pathway from the respiratory center in the brain stem, the cervical spinal cord, and neuromuscular disease as well as restrictive disorders preventing lung expansion, such as pleural space disease; or, rarely, severe primary pulmonary disease such as pneumonia. The most common cause of hypoventilation in perioperative patients is depression of the respiratory center from anesthetics and/or analgesics, but it can also be caused by upper airway obstruction, especially in brachycephalic breeds, as well as neurologic impairment in postoperative cervical intervertebral disc disease, cervical spinal fracture repairs, or craniotomies. Treatment is designed to correct the underlying problem. If respiratory center depression is the cause and the patient is under anesthesia, positive pressure ventilation is indicated. In the postoperative period, partial reversal of the anesthetic drugs may be sufficient to correct the hypoventilation. Neurologic causes may also require positive pressure ventilation (oxygenation and ventilation are discussed by Rozanski elsewhere in this issue). Venous admixture, the third cause of hypoxemia, occurs when venous blood moves from the right to the left side of the circulation without being appropriately oxygenated. In perioperative patients, this commonly occurs secondary to atelectasis from small airway and alveolar collapse. Supplemental oxygen should be provided to these patients, and postoperative patients should be turned regularly and encouraged to stand and walk to attempt to recruit collapsed alveoli. Also, during prolonged anesthesia times, medical air can be used instead of 100% oxygen to reduce the risk of absorption atelectasis.[34]

POSTOPERATIVE DERANGEMENTS
Hypernatremia

Central diabetes insipidus (CDI) results from partial or complete lack of vasopressin production from the neurohypophysis.[1] Although CDI is most common in veterinary patients with intracranial disease, it can also been seen secondary to hypoxic or ischemic encephalopathy following trauma, severe shock, or after cardiopulmonary arrest causing decreased antidiuretic hormone (ADH) release.[35–38] This cause of CDI is usually transient, but it can result in significant hypernatremia in postoperative patients.[39] These patients have increased serum sodium concentrations and osmolality, and usually have hyposthenuric urine (unless severely dehydrated, in which case they may approach isosthenuria). Clinical experience indicates that this is most common in postoperative gastric dilatation-volvulus cases, but other surgical cases, including gastrointestinal resection and anastomosis, septic peritonitis, hemoabdomen, and occasionally thoracotomy, may also be affected. These patients are often administered high rates of sodium-rich fluids, such as Normosol-R, Plasmalyte-A, or LRS, often with hetastarch, which is most commonly administered in 0.9% NaCl. Most patients with normal renal function are able to handle the high sodium load that is provided by this type of fluid administration, and as the serum sodium concentration and osmolality increase, the patients have increased thirst. The increased intake of free water corrects the serum sodium concentration and osmolality. However, in postoperative patients that may be unable or unwilling to drink right away, severe hypernatremia may result.

Before a treatment plan for hypernatremia is instituted, the patient's volume status must be assessed. If the patient is hypovolemic and hypernatremic, then volume expansion should occur with isotonic fluids. The degree of hypernatremia helps determine which fluid is most appropriate. With mild hypernatremia, Normosol-R or Plasmalyte-A (sodium concentration of approximately 145 mEq/L) may be reasonable choices. If the patient is moderately hypernatremic, then 0.9% NaCl is a better choice because of its higher sodium concentration (154 mEq/L). More commonly, these postoperative patients are euvolemic, because they have already had adequate fluid resuscitation. Although the lack of ADH causes water loss, it is usually not to the degree that they become hypovolemic because they are on concurrent IV fluid therapy. The patient's free water deficit can be calculated using the equation[40]:

$$\text{Free water deficit (L)} = (\text{current } [Na^+]/\text{normal } [Na^+] - 1) \times [0.6 \times \text{body weight (kg)}]$$

This equation gives the total volume of free water that should be replaced, and can be given over the number of hours that have been calculated to be needed to safely reduce the sodium concentration (typically 0.5 mEq/L/h or 10–12 mEq/L/d) if the hypernatremia is chronic, although this is rarely a concern in postoperative patients. Too-rapid correction of hypernatremia can result in cellular swelling and neuronal edema and can lead to life-threatening neurologic complications. Treatment of these patients is designed to increase free water to reduce the sodium concentration. If the patient is willing and able to drink, providing access to small amounts of water divided incrementally may be sufficient therapy. In more severe cases in which serum sodium concentration is rapidly increasing (>160 mmol/L) and the patient is not drinking, water loss can be replaced with 5% dextrose, which is given along with a maintenance rate of isotonic fluids (2 mL/kg/h). Alternatively, 5% dextrose at a rate of 3.7 mL/kg/h can be given along with maintenance isotonic fluids, and this usually reduces the sodium concentration at the desired rate in dogs.[28] This protocol is contraindicated in patients that cannot tolerate high fluid rates, and should only be used in patients in which frequent measurement (every 2–4 hours) of sodium concentration can be performed.

The most common complication of hypernatremia therapy is neuronal and cerebral edema. If a patient shows neurologic signs such as a change in mental status, seizures, head-pressing or other disorders of behavior or movement, fluid therapy should be stopped immediately and serum sodium should be rechecked. A decrease in measured sodium level in combination with neurologic signs should prompt treatment of cerebral edema, which may include mannitol (0.5–1 g/kg IV over 20–30 minutes) or hypertonic saline (7.2% solution at 3–5 mL/kg over 20 minutes).[40]

An additional treatment that may be indicated in severe cases of hypernatremia secondary to CDI is the administration of exogenous ADH. If the patient has CDI, vasopressin or desmopressin can be used to control the sodium. Desmopressin acetate can be given at a dose of 1 to 2 drops in both eyes every 12 to 24 hours.[1] Careful monitoring of both the patient's sodium concentration and body weight should occur to prevent rapid changes. Fluid therapy may need to be adjusted as well, particularly if large amounts of free water were being administered. Exogenous ADH and fluids containing free water can cause rapid and dangerous decreases in sodium concentration and plasma osmolality.

Renal Tubular Acidosis

Renal tubular acidosis (RTA) is associated with a metabolic acidosis caused by either decreased sodium bicarbonate reabsorption (proximal RTA or type 2) or a lack of hydrogen ion excretion (distal RTA or type 1).[41] Type 1 RTA can occur secondary to marked volume depletion or urinary tract obstruction, and so can become evident in postoperative patients.[42] The diagnosis of type 1 RTA can be made when there is an increased urine pH (>6.0) with a concurrent metabolic acidosis, providing that a urinary tract infection with a urease-positive organism has been ruled out. RTA should be suspected in cases that have a persistent metabolic acidosis that is not secondary to more common causes such as lactic acidosis, uremia, ketoacidosis, severe diarrhea, or exogenous acids (ethylene glycol). Evaluation of the anion gap is helpful, because the anion gap is normal in cases with RTA and diarrhea, and increased in all other causes of metabolic acidosis.

Treatment of RTA depends on the severity of the metabolic acidosis. Mild cases with minimal effect on the blood pH may be self-limiting and not require any therapy. More severe cases may benefit from the administration of sodium bicarbonate. There are several potential risks of sodium bicarbonate therapy, and administration should only be considered when necessary. Risks include hypercapnia and paradoxic cerebral acidosis, hypokalemia and ionized hypocalcemia, hypernatremia, hypervolemia, and hyperosmolality. Dosing is based on the following equation: mEq of sodium bicarbonate = 0.3 × body weight (kg) × base deficit. Usually one-quarter to one-third of the dose is given over 4 to 6 hours. Because sodium bicarbonate is hypertonic, is must be diluted to an osmolality of less than 600 mOsm/L before peripheral administration. For the commercially available sodium bicarbonate (8.4%), its osmolality is roughly 2000 mOsm/L, and hence it should be diluted at least 1:3 with sterile water for administration through a peripheral catheter.[43] This dilution is particularly important in patients that are hypernatremic concurrently, because the sodium load provided by the bicarbonate is significant. However, RTA secondary to severe hypovolemia is a transient disease process, so repeat dosing of sodium bicarbonate is not usually needed while hospitalized, and no long-term therapy is necessary.

SUMMARY

Correction of acid-base and electrolyte disturbances is crucial for optimal outcome in perioperative patients. A thorough physical examination and close monitoring are key in recognition and treatment of many of the most common disorders discussed earlier, and the importance of serial examinations cannot be overemphasized in these dynamic patients. Cardiovascular and respiratory failure and death may result if acid-base and electrolyte disturbances are not promptly recognized and treated appropriately.

REFERENCES

1. DiBartola SP. Introduction to acid–base disorders. In: DiBartola SP, editor. Fluid, electrolyte, and acid–base disorders in small animal practice. 4th ed. St. Louis: Elsevier Saunders; 2012. p. 231–52.
2. Middleton DJ, Ilkiw JE, Watson ADJ. Arterial and venous blood gas tensions in clinically healthy cats. Am J Vet Res 1981;42:1609–11.
3. Pang DS, Boysen S. Lactate in veterinary critical care: pathophysiology and management. J Am Anim Hosp Assoc 2007;43:270–9.
4. Shapiro BA, Peruzzi WT. Interpretation of blood gases. In: Ayres SM, Grenvik A, Holbrook PR, et al, editors. Textbook of critical care. 3rd edition. Philadelphia: WB Saunders; 1995. p. 278–94.
5. Lagutchik MS, Ogilvie GK, Wingfield WE, et al. Lactate kinetics in veterinary critical care: a review. J Vet Emerg Crit Care 1996;6(2):81–95.
6. Luft FC. Lactic acidosis update for critical care clinicians. J Am Soc Nephrol 2001;12:S15–9.
7. Allen SE, Holm JL. Lactate: physiology and clinical utility. J Vet Emerg Crit Care 2008;18(2):123–32.
8. Sharkey LC, Wellman ML. Use of lactate in small animal clinical practice. Vet Clin Small Anim 2013;43:1287–97.
9. Lagutchik MS. Lactate. In: Vade SL, Knoll JS, Smith FW, et al, editors. Blackwell's five minute veterinary consult: laboratory tests and diagnostic procedures. Ames (IA): Wiley-Blackwell; 2009. p. 388–9.
10. Rand JS, Kinnaird E, Baglioni A, et al. Acute stress hyperglycemia in cats is associated with struggling and increased concentrations of lactate and norepinephrine. J Vet Intern Med 2002;16(2):123–32.
11. Redavid LA, Sharp CR, Mitchell MA, et al. Plasma lactate measurement in healthy cats. J Vet Emerg Crit Care 2012;22:123–32.
12. Aslar AK, Kuzu MA, Elhan AH, et al. Admission lactate level and the APACHE II are the most useful predictors of prognosis following torso trauma. Injury 2004; 35(8):746–52.
13. Bakker J, Coffernils M, Leon M, et al. Blood lactate levels are superior to oxygen-derived variables in predicting outcome in human septic shock. Chest 1991;99: 956–62.
14. Bernardin G, Pradier C, Tiger F, et al. Blood pressure and arterial lactate level are early indicators of short-term survival in human septic shock. Intensive Care Med 1996;22:17–25.

15. Nguyen HB, Rivers EP, Knoblich BP, et al. Early lactate clearance is associated with improved outcome in severe sepsis and septic shock. Crit Care Med 2004;32(8):1637–42.
16. Abramson D, Scalea T, Hitchcock R, et al. Lactate clearance and survival following injury. J Trauma 1993;35(4):584–9.
17. Arnold RC, Shapiro NI, Jones AE, et al. Multicenter study of early lactate clearance as a determinant of survival in patients with presumed sepsis. Shock 2009;32(1):35–9.
18. McNelis J, Marini C, Jurkiewicz A, et al. Prolonged lactate clearance is associated with increased mortality in the surgical intensive care unit. Am J Surg 2001;182:481–5.
19. Beer KA, Syring RS, Drobatz KJ. Evaluation of plasma lactate concentration and base excess at the time of hospital admission as predictors of gastric necrosis and outcome and correlation between those variables in dogs with gastric dilatation-volvulus: 78 cases (2004–2009). J Am Vet Med Assoc 2013;242:54–8.
20. de Papp E, Drobatz KJ, Hughes D. Plasma lactate concentration as a predictor of gastric necrosis and survival among dogs with gastric dilatation-volvulus: 102 cases (1995–1998). J Am Vet Med Assoc 1999;215(1):49–52.
21. Green TI, Tonozzi CC, Kirby R, et al. Evaluation of initial plasma lactate values as a predictor of gastric necrosis and initial and subsequent plasma lactate values as a predictor of survival in dogs with gastric dilatation-volvulus: 84 dogs (2003–2007). J Vet Emerg Crit Care 2011;21:36–44.
22. Holahan ML, Brown AJ, Drobatz KJ. The associated of blood lactate concentration with outcome in dogs with idiopathic immune-mediated hemolytic anemia: 173 cases. J Vet Emerg Crit Care 2010;20:413–20.
23. Nel M, Lobetti RG, Kellen N, et al. Prognostic value of blood lactate, blood glucose and hematocrit in canine babesiosis. J Vet Intern Med 2004;18(4):471–6.
24. Zacher LA, Verg J, Shaw SP, et al. Association between outcome and changes in plasma lactate concentration during presurgical treatment in dogs with gastric dilatation-volvulus: 64 cases. J Am Vet Med Assoc 2010;236:892–7.
25. Kelm DJ, Perrin JT, Cartin-Ceba R, et al. Fluid overload in patients with severe sepsis and septic shock treated with early goal-directed therapy is associated with increased acute need for fluid-related medical interventions and hospital death. Shock 2015;43(1):68–73.
26. Schaer M. Hyperkalemia in cats with urethral obstruction: electrocardiographs abnormalities and treatment. Vet Clin North Am 1977;7(2):407–14.
27. Tag TL, Day TK. Electrocardiographic assessment of hyperkalemia in dogs and cats. J Vet Emerg Crit Care 2008;18(1):61–7.
28. Pascoe PJ. Perioperative management of fluid therapy. In: DiBartola SP, editor. Fluid, electrolyte, and acid-base disorders in small animal practice. 4th edition. St Louis (MO): Elsevier Saunders; 2012. p. 391–419.
29. Riordan L, Schaer M. Potassium disorders. In: Silverstein DC, Hopper K, editors. Small animal critical care medicine. 2nd edition. St Louis (MO): Elsevier; 2015. p. 269–73.
30. Drobatz KJ, Cole SG. The influence of crystalloid type on acid-base and electrolyte status of cats with urethral obstruction. J Vet Emerg Crit Care 2008;18(4):355–61.
31. Boag AK, Coe RJ, Matinez TA, et al. Acid-base and electrolyte abnormalities in dogs with gastrointestinal foreign bodies. J Vet Intern Med 2005;19(6):816–21.
32. Ha YS, Hopper K, Epstein SE. Incidence, nature and etiology of metabolic alkalosis in dogs cats. J Vet Intern Med 2013;27(4):847–53.

33. Haskins SC. Hypoxemia. In: Silverstein DC, Hopper K, editors. Small animal critical care medicine. 2nd edition. St Louis (MO): Elsevier; 2015. p. 81–6.
34. O'Brien J. Absorption atelectasis: incidence and clinical implications. AANA J 2013;81(3):205–8.
35. Aroch I, Mazaki-Tovi M, Shemesh O, et al. Central diabetes insipidus in five cats: clinical presentation, diagnosis and oral desmopressin therapy. J Feline Med Surg 2005;7:333.
36. Harb MF, Nelson RW, Feldman EC, et al. Central diabetes insipidus in dogs: 20 cases (1986–1995). J Am Vet Med Assoc 1996;209:1884.
37. Leaf A. Neurogenic diabetes insipidus. Kidney Int 1979;5:572.
38. Wickramasinge LS, Chazan BJ, Mandal AR, et al. CDI after upper GI hemorrhage. Br Med J (Clin Res Ed) 1988;296:969.
39. Herrod PJ, Awad S, Redfern A, et al. Hypo- and hypernatremia in surgical patients: is there room for improvement? World J Surg 2010;34:495–9.
40. Burkitt Creedon JM. Sodium disorders. In: Silverstein DC, Hopper K, editors. Small animal critical care medicine. 2nd edition. St Louis (MO): Elsevier; 2015. p. 263–8.
41. Riordan L, Schaer M. Renal tubular acidosis. Compend Contin Educ Vet 2005;27: 513–28.
42. Kurtzman NA. Renal tubular acidosis: a constellation of syndromes. Hosp Pract 1987;22(11):131.
43. Hopper K. Traditional acid-base analysis. In: Silverstein DC, Hopper K, editors. Small animal critical care medicine. 2nd edition. St Louis (MO): Elsevier; 2015. p. 289–95.

Perioperative Monitoring of Heart Rate and Rhythm

Mark A. Oyama, DVM

KEYWORDS

- Arrhythmia • Antiarrhythmics • Electrocardiography

KEY POINTS

- When assessing perioperative arrhythmias, it is important to obtain an accurate electrocardiographic diagnosis, assess patient hemodynamic status during the arrhythmia, and determine whether underlying primary cardiac disease is present.
- The decision on whether to treat a specific arrhythmia should be based on the presence or absence of hemodynamic signs and risk of sudden death.
- If antiarrhythmic therapy is deemed necessary, consider the likely mechanisms of arrhythmia, address transient imbalances that contribute to arrhythmia formation, and select antiarrhythmic agents based on mechanism of action and arrhythmia diagnosis.
- Whether or not treatment is initiated, continuous and careful monitoring of electrocardiogram rhythm and hemodynamics is advisable.

NATURE OF THE PROBLEM
Introduction

Disorders of heart rate and rhythms in the perioperative period are common and can occur in animals with or without underlying primary cardiac or conduction system disease. Primary cardiac diseases that are associated with high baseline risk for clinically important arrhythmias include myocardial diseases such as hypertrophic, dilated, and arrhythmogenic cardiomyopathy; pericardial disorders; conduction system diseases such as sick sinus syndrome or atrioventricular (AV) nodal block; and, to a lesser extent, myxomatous mitral valve disease. Observational studies reveal that perioperative arrhythmias are commonly encountered in noncardiac conditions (**Box 1**) such as gastric dilatation-volvulus (GDV), hemoabdomen, and splenic mass, wherein the incidence of ventricular arrhythmias is 50.6% to 77.4%,[1,2] 32%,[3] and 28.4%,[4] respectively. Some of these studies indicate that the presence of perioperative arrhythmias is associated with an increase in mortality,[3,4] whereas others do not.[1] Although these observational studies provide evidence that perioperative arrhythmias are a common

Disclosure: The author has nothing to disclose.
Department of Clinical Studies, Matthew J. Ryan Veterinary Hospital, University of Pennsylvania, School of Veterinary Medicine, 3900 Delancey Street, Philadelphia, PA 19104, USA
E-mail address: maoyama@vet.upenn.edu

Vet Clin Small Anim 45 (2015) 953–963
http://dx.doi.org/10.1016/j.cvsm.2015.04.002   **vetsmall.theclinics.com**
0195-5616/15/$ – see front matter © 2015 Elsevier Inc. All rights reserved.

Box 1
Diseases commonly associated with perioperative arrhythmias

- Splenic or hepatic masses or neoplasia
- Gastric dilatation and volvulus
- Pericardial disease requiring pericardiectomy
- Pulmonary disease requiring lung lobectomy
- Pulmonic stenosis undergoing balloon valvuloplasty

---

clinical occurrence, they are unable to indicate whether intervention to suppress these arrhythmias improves outcome. In one retrospective study of dogs undergoing surgery for GDV, prophylactic perioperative lidocaine administration was not associated with reduced mortality.[5] Important aspects of the problem include the following:

- Perioperative cardiac arrhythmias are common.
- Their effect on morbidity and mortality is largely unknown.
- The benefit in treating or not treating perioperative arrhythmias is likely influenced by many different factors including the following:
  - Presence or absence of underlying primary cardiac disease
  - Presence or absence of underlying extracardiac disease
  - Nature of the cardiac arrhythmia (eg, rhythm, rate, frequency)
  - Presence or absence of aggravating factors or transient physiologic imbalances (discussed later)
- The precise effect of these and other factors in overall survival is unknown, which makes decision making around when and what to treat extremely difficult.

Mechanisms of Arrhythmia Formation

Arrhythmias arise from disorders of impulse formation or conduction (**Box 2**). Injury to cardiac tissue and arrhythmogenesis can occur from a variety of insults, including ischemia, fibrosis, inflammation, necrosis, or oxidative stress. In many patients with perioperative arrhythmias, the exact nature of the cardiac injury is unknown. Careful inspection of the electrocardiogram (ECG) and cardiac blood tests such as cardiac

---

Box 2
Mechanisms of arrhythmogenesis and examples of commonly associated arrhythmias

- Disorders of impulse formation
  - Enhanced or suppressed normal automaticity: examples include sinus bradycardia, sinus arrest, sinus tachycardia, accelerated junctional or ventricular escape rhythms.
  - Abnormal automaticity: examples include supraventricular or ventricular premature beats or tachycardia.
  - Triggered activity (early or late afterdepolarizations): examples include supraventricular or ventricular premature beats or tachycardia.
- Disorders of impulse conduction
  - Bundle branch blocks: examples include right or left bundle branch block, which do not require treatment in the absence of other arrhythmias or ECG abnormalities.
  - Reentry circuits: examples include supraventricular or ventricular premature beats or tachycardia.

---

troponin-I might help identify likely causes. For instance, ST segment depression and increased cardiac troponin-I level are suggestive of myocardial ischemia and necrosis.

Role of Transient Imbalances

The importance of transient imbalances in the genesis of perioperative arrhythmias is well accepted.[6] Transient imbalances are temporary circumstances that provide a substrate for arrhythmia formation and lead to the development or worsening of arrhythmias (**Box 3**). Transient imbalances in the presence of cardiac injury might be sufficient to lead to life-threatening arrhythmias. Identification and treatment of such imbalances plays an important role in the management of perioperative arrhythmias such that removal of transient imbalances could be all that is needed to reduce the incidence or severity of arrhythmia formation.

APPROACH TO MANAGEMENT
Diagnosis of Perioperative Arrhythmias

A complete review of ECG evaluation is beyond the scope of this article and the reader is referred to a variety of excellent sources for additional information.[7–9] Several of the most important ECG characteristics of perioperative arrhythmias are listed in **Box 4**.

Decision to Treat

The decision of when to treat perioperative arrhythmias (**Fig. 1**) is depends on the answer to the following 2 questions:

- Are there clinical signs caused by altered hemodynamics during the arrhythmia?
- Does the arrhythmia predispose to a high risk of sudden arrhythmic death (ie, ventricular fibrillation)?

Box 3
Partial list of transient imbalances that promote arrhythmogenesis

- Autonomic imbalance
  - Increased sympathetic tone caused by stress, pain, sympathomimetic drugs.
  - Increased parasympathetic tone caused by gastrointestinal, respiratory, or central nervous system disease; opioids; parasympathomimetic drugs; laryngoscopy; or tracheal intubation.
- Electrolyte or metabolic disturbances
  - Hyperkalemia caused by urinary obstruction, hypoadrenocorticism, renal failure, drugs, acidosis.
  - Hypokalemia caused by vomiting, diarrhea, polyuria, diuresis, drugs.
  - Metabolic acidosis caused by poor tissue perfusion, toxins, diabetic ketoacidosis, diarrhea.
  - Respiratory acidosis caused by inadequate ventilation, pulmonary disease, poor cardiac output.
- Myocardial ischemia caused by poor cardiac output, structural heart disease, thromboembolism, hypoxemia, anemia.
- Indwelling catheters or devices such as pacemakers, tracheal tubes, central venous or pulmonary artery catheters, chest tubes.
- Systemic derangements associated with inflammation, cytokine release, sepsis, myocarditis, paraneoplastic syndromes.

Box 4
Important electrocardiographic characteristics of perioperative arrhythmias

- Heart rate: what is the heart rate of the arrhythmia? Arrhythmias with rates greater than 180 bpm (dog) or greater than 220 bpm (cat) or less than 50 bpm (dog) or less than 90 bpm (cat) tend to be associated with increased risk for clinical signs.

- Frequency: how often does the arrhythmia occur? Frequent or sustained (>30 seconds in duration) arrhythmias tend to be more associated with clinical signs.

- Origin of beats: are the ectopic beats originating from or above the AV node (supraventricular origin) or from the ventricle (ventricular origin)? Ventricular origin beats tend to be more associated with a high risk for hemodynamic compromise or sudden death versus supraventricular origin beats.

- AV synchrony: is synchrony between atrial and ventricular contraction maintained? Loss of AV synchrony is associated with greater risk for significant reduction in cardiac output. Examples of ECG rhythms with loss of AV synchrony include ventricular tachycardia, complete AV nodal block, and atrial fibrillation.

Patients with findings related to poor hemodynamics, such as hypotension, weakness, syncope, poor tissue perfusion, congestion, and hypothermia, benefit from interventions to correct the arrhythmia. In the absence of clinical findings indicating poor hemodynamics, the decision to treat is based on whether the arrhythmia is thought likely to degenerate into a clinically significant or fatal arrhythmia. Unlike the former indication, the decision to treat based on future risk of signs or sudden death is often extremely difficult to make. The following criteria are often used as indicators of increased risk for sudden death and triggers to begin treatment:

- Heart rate: rates greater than 180 beats per minute (bpm) (dog) or greater than 220 bpm (cat) or less than 50 bpm (dog) or less than 90 bpm (cat) tend to be associated with increased risk for clinical signs
- Sustained versus nonsustained arrhythmias: those persisting for more than 30 seconds at a time tend to be more associated with increased risk for clinical signs
- R-on-T phenomenon: single or multiple premature beats with rapid rates wherein the R wave of the ectopic beat encroaches on the preceding beat's T wave are considered to signal increased risk for malignant ventricular arrhythmias
- Presence of underlying structural heart disease: in particular, those diseases such as dilated, hypertrophic, restrictive, or arrhythmogenic cardiomyopathy that tend to be associated with electrical instability and sudden death
- Cardiac troponin-I: markedly increased serum or plasma concentrations tend to be associated with more severe myocardial injury and dysfunction

Arrhythmias that commonly cause hemodynamic compromise include the following:

- Rapid and sustained supraventricular or ventricular tachycardia
- High-grade second-degree AV nodal block
- Third-degree or complete AV nodal block
- Sinus arrest greater than 4 seconds
- Atrial fibrillation with rapid ventricular heart rate (>160–180 bpm)

These arrhythmias might require treatment because of their effects on hemodynamics regardless of the risk for development of ventricular fibrillation. In general,

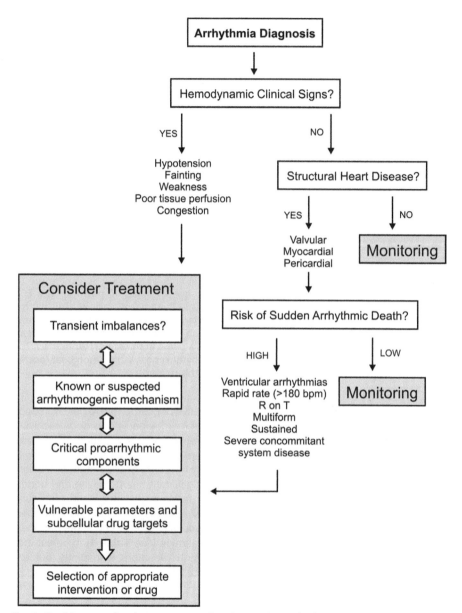

Fig. 1. Decision tree for the treatment of perioperative arrhythmias. See text for details.

arrhythmias that commonly do not require specific antiarrhythmic treatment include the following:

- Infrequent supraventricular or ventricular premature beats
- Accelerated ventricular escape rhythms (slow ventricular tachycardia) (**Fig. 2**)
- First-degree AV nodal block
- Infrequent second-degree AV nodal block
- Sinus arrest less than 2 seconds
- Atrial fibrillation with slow ventricular heart rate (<160–180 bpm)

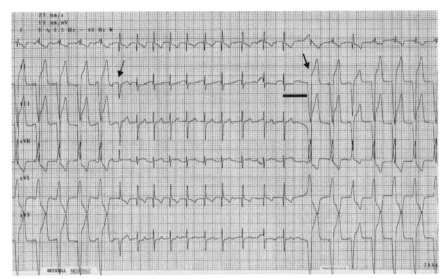

Fig. 2. Six-lead ECG from a dog following splenectomy (25 mm/s; 10 mm/mV). The ECG shows an accelerated (idioventricular) ventricular escape rhythm (*solid arrow*). This rhythm is differentiated from ventricular tachycardia by its slow rate (approximately 130 bpm) and the timing of its onset, which is more consistent with an escape beat than a premature beat. Note that the ectopic ventricular rhythm begins after a pause in the sinus rhythm (*bar*). The preceding episode of accelerated ventricular escape rhythm ends with a fusion beat (*dotted arrow*), which is a common finding in patients with this rhythm.

Development of atrial fibrillation in the intraoperative or postoperative period in dogs with normal underlying myocardial function is common, especially in dogs receiving anesthetic or pain control medications that increase vagal tone, such as opioids. Increased parasympathetic tone to atrial myocardium increases the heterogeneity of refractoriness, which predisposes to develop of primary or lone atrial fibrillation. In contrast with atrial fibrillation in animals with significant heart disease and underlying atrial enlargement, primary atrial fibrillation tends to produce slow ventricular rates and is often self-limiting and spontaneously resolves once the offending drug is reduced or discontinued. The author has had success in converting acute perioperative atrial fibrillation with intravenous (IV) procainamide (see **Table 1**) in canine patients. Other drugs, such as IV amiodarone, might be more efficacious but are associated with a high risk of adverse side effects.[10,11]

Therapeutic Options

Therapeutic options include supportive measures and interventions to address transient imbalances as well as administration of antiarrhythmic drugs. Included in the supportive measures and interventions are the following:

- Removal of offending drugs
- Correction of acid-base status
- Correction of electrolyte derangements
- Correction of hypoxemia
- Correction of low cardiac perfusion
- Correction of hemostatic disorders
- Correction of device placement

- Reduction of stress or pain
- Correction of inflammatory or septic processes

If drug-based antiarrhythmic therapy is initiated, as much as possible, the specific antiarrhythmic is chosen based on the suspected mechanisms of arrhythmogenesis and identification of critical proarrhythmogenic components, vulnerable parameters, and subcellular drug targets (**Fig. 3**). The goal of therapy in patients with compromised hemodynamics is to improve cardiac output and tissue perfusion and alleviate any signs of congestion rather than complete suppression of the offending arrhythmia. Overly aggressive drug administration based on the ECG rhythm alone can predispose to adverse side effects, including proarrhythmia. The goal of therapy in patients at risk for sudden death is to normalize the myocardial electrical environment and increase the threshold for ventricular fibrillation. A list of common drugs used for therapy for perioperative arrhythmias is presented in **Table 1**. Initiation of drug therapy is accompanied by monitoring of ECG rhythm and hemodynamic status. In instances in which the mechanism of arrhythmogenesis is unclear or could have a variety of causes, empiric drug therapy based on the ECG diagnosis alone is attempted.

MONITORING AND CLINICAL OUTCOMES

The optimal clinical outcome of perioperative arrhythmias is return to normal sinus rhythm; however, as previously mentioned, some arrhythmias are well tolerated and might not require any (further) treatment. Monitoring of patients receiving antiarrhythmic therapy can include any or all of the following:

- Continuous or frequent ECG monitoring
- Echocardiography
- Blood pressure measurement
- Respiratory rate and effort
- Lactate concentration
- Acid-base and electrolyte status
- Cardiac troponin-I concentration

In some patients, a single or limited number of IV boluses of antiarrhythmic agents might be sufficient to suppress important arrhythmias as transient imbalances resolve. In other patients, constant-rate infusions of agents might be needed in the perioperative period for more sustained control of arrhythmias, and, in some cases, longerterm continuation of oral antiarrhythmic therapy might be indicated beyond hospital discharge. Arrhythmias are often sporadic, and assessment of whether or not a drug is effectively controlling both clinical signs and ECG rhythm after discharge requires close monitoring by the owner as well as frequent ECG rechecks or 24-hour ambulatory ECG (Holter) monitoring. In patients that are recovering well in the postoperative period, gradual weaning of IV or oral antiarrhythmics is performed in the hopes that return to health and resolution of transient imbalances render long-term antiarrhythmic therapy unnecessary.

Cardiac troponin-I is released by cardiac myocytes in proportion to cellular damage and necrosis. Increased circulating concentrations have been reported in dogs and cats with a wide variety of both cardiac and noncardiac diseases, including cardiomyopathy, valve disease, myocarditis, pericardial effusion, GDV, pulmonary disease, trauma, heat stroke, and hemoabdomen. In patients with heart disease[12] or systemic inflammation,[13,14] increased cardiac troponin-I level is associated with decreased survival. In general, markedly increased or increasing cardiac troponin-I concentrations are seen as evidence of ongoing myocardial injury and potential for electrical

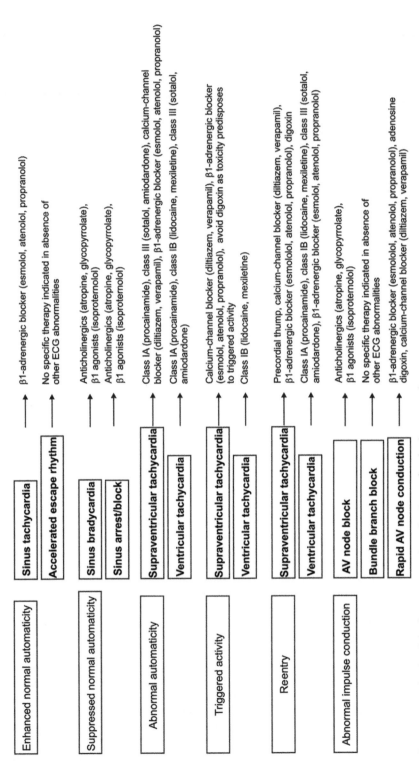

Fig. 3. Drug selection based on suspected mechanisms of arrhythmogenesis.

Table 1
Common drugs used for the treatment of perioperative arrhythmias in dogs and cats

Atenolol	Dog: 0.25–2.0 mg/kg PO q12–24 h Cat: 6.25–12.5 mg PO q12–24 h
Atropine sulfate	Dog and cat: 0.01–0.04 mg/kg IV, IM, SC, prn
Diltiazem	Dog: 0.5–2 mg/kg PO q8 h; 0.1–0.2 mg/kg IV bolus, then 2–6 µg/kg/min IV CRI Cat: 1.0–2.5 mg/kg PO q8 h; 0.1–0.2 mg/kg IV bolus, then 2–6 µg/kg/min IV CRI. Sustained-release diltiazem: Dilacor XR: 30–60 mg PO q24 h
Esmolol	Dog and cat: 50–100 µg/kg IV bolus every 5 min (up to 500 µg/kg max), then 25–200 µg/kg/min CRI
Glycopyrrolate	Dog and cat: 0.005–0.01 mg/kg IV, IM; 0.01–0.02 mg/kg SC
Isoproterenol	Dog and cat: 0.04–0.09 µg/kg/min IV; 10 µg/kg IM, SC q6 h
Lidocaine	Dog: 2 mg/kg slowly IV, interosseous (double the dose if given intratracheally) up to 3 boluses, then 30–80 µg/kg/min CRI Cat: 0.25–0.75 mg/kg IV over 5 min (use with caution because seizures can develop)
Mexiletine	Dog: 4–8 mg/kg PO q8–12 h
Procainamide	Dog: 2 mg/kg IV over 3–5 min up to total dose of 15 mg/kg, then 25–50 µg/kg/min CRI; 10–30 mg/kg IM, PO q6 h Cat: 2–5 mg/kg PO q6–8 h
Propranolol	Dog: 0.02–0.06 mg/kg IV over 5–10 min; 0.2–1.0 mg/kg PO q8 h Cat <4.5 kg: 0.02–0.06 mg/kg IV over 5–10 min; 2.5–5 mg PO q8–12 h. Cat >4.5 kg: 5 mg PO 8–12 h
Quinidine gluconate	Dog: 6–20 mg/kg PO, IM q6 h; 6–20 mg/kg PO q8 h with sustained-release products
Quinidine sulfate	Dog: 5–10 mg/kg IV (very slowly)
Sotalol	Dog: 1–2 mg/kg PO q12 h Cat: 10 mg PO q12 h
Verapamil	Dog: 0.05 mg/kg slow IV (1–2 min) boluses given at intervals of 10–30 min (to effect) to a maximum cumulative dose of 0.2 mg/kg Cat: 0.05 mg/kg slow IV, may repeat twice as described for dog

Abbreviations: CRI, constant rate infusion; IM, intramuscular; PO, orally; prn, as needed; q, every; SC, subcutaneous.

instability, whereas decreasing concentrations suggest an acute injury that is resolving. The half-life of cardiac troponin-I in the dog is short and serial (daily or weekly) monitoring might help inform the need for antiarrhythmic therapy; however, further studies of the relationship between cardiac troponin-I and outcome in patients with perioperative arrhythmias are needed.

COMPLICATIONS AND CONCERNS

Complications of antiarrhythmic therapy for perioperative arrhythmias can include hypotension, central nervous system signs, proarrhythmia, exacerbation of congestion, or gastrointestinal signs, depending on the specific antiarrhythmic agent. During therapy, continuous ECG monitoring and either continuous or frequent blood pressure monitoring is recommended. If transient imbalances are identified and addressed, frequent reassessment for their reoccurrence is performed. As the patient recovers from its operative procedure, gradual withdrawal of antiarrhythmic agents is attempted. Long-term antiarrhythmic therapy is seldom required in patients with normal underlying cardiac structure. Persistent, refractory, or worsening arrhythmias might signal the presence of underlying cardiac injury or disease, and further diagnostics, such as radiographs or echocardiography, should be considered.

SUMMARY

When assessing perioperative arrhythmias, it is important to obtain an accurate electrocardiographic diagnosis, assess patient hemodynamic status during the arrhythmia, and determine whether underlying primary cardiac disease is present. The decision on whether to treat a specific arrhythmia should be based on the presence or absence of hemodynamic signs and risk of sudden death. If antiarrhythmic therapy is deemed necessary, consider the likely mechanisms of arrhythmia, address transient imbalances that contribute to arrhythmia formation, and select antiarrhythmic agents based on mechanism of action and arrhythmia diagnosis. Whether or not treatment is initiated, continuous and careful monitoring of ECG rhythm and hemodynamics is advisable.

REFERENCES

1. Beck JJ, Staatz AJ, Pelsue DH, et al. Risk factors associated with short-term outcome and development of perioperative complications in dogs undergoing surgery because of gastric dilatation-volvulus: 166 cases (1992-2003). J Am Vet Med Assoc 2006;229(12):1934–9.
2. Mackenzie G, Barnhart M, Kennedy S, et al. A retrospective study of factors influencing survival following surgery for gastric dilatation-volvulus syndrome in 306 dogs. J Am Anim Hosp Assoc 2010;46(2):97–102.
3. Lux CN, Culp WT, Mayhew PD, et al. Perioperative outcome in dogs with hemoperitoneum: 83 cases (2005-2010). J Am Vet Med Assoc 2013;242(10):1385–91.
4. Wendelburg KM, O'Toole TE, McCobb E, et al. Risk factors for perioperative death in dogs undergoing splenectomy for splenic masses: 539 cases (2001-2012). J Am Vet Med Assoc 2014;245(12):1382–90.
5. Buber T, Saragusty J, Ranen E, et al. Evaluation of lidocaine treatment and risk factors for death associated with gastric dilatation and volvulus in dogs: 112 cases (1997-2005). J Am Vet Med Assoc 2007;230(9):1334–9.
6. Atlee JL. Perioperative cardiac dysrhythmias: diagnosis and management. Anesthesiology 1997;86(6):1397–424.
7. Oyama MA, Kraus MS, Gelzer AR. Rapid review of ECG interpretation in small animal practice. Boca Raton (FL): CRC Press; 2013.
8. Martin M. Small animal ECGs: an introductory guide. Hoboken (NJ): Wiley-Blackwell; 2007.
9. Tilley LP, Burtnick N. ECGs for the small animal practitioner (Made Easy series). Jackson (WY): Teton New Media; 2009.
10. Oyama MA, Prosek R. Acute conversion of atrial fibrillation in two dogs by intravenous amiodarone administration. J Vet Intern Med 2006;20(5):1224–7.
11. Cober RE, Schober KE, Hildebrandt N, et al. Adverse effects of intravenous amiodarone in 5 dogs. J Vet Intern Med 2009;23(3):657–61.
12. Hezzell MJ, Boswood A, Chang YM, et al. The combined prognostic potential of serum high-sensitivity cardiac troponin I and N-terminal pro-B-type natriuretic peptide concentrations in dogs with degenerative mitral valve disease. J Vet Intern Med 2012;26(2):302–11.

13. Langhorn R, Oyama MA, King LG, et al. Prognostic importance of myocardial injury in critically ill dogs with systemic inflammation. J Vet Intern Med 2013; 27(4):895–903.
14. Hamacher L, Dorfelt R, Muller M, et al. Serum cardiac troponin I concentrations in dogs with systemic inflammatory response syndrome. J Vet Intern Med 2015; 29(1):164–70.

Perioperative Blood Pressure Control and Management

Tanya Duke-Novakovski, BVetMed, MSc, DVA,
Anthony Carr, Dr med vet*

KEYWORDS

- Blood pressure • Anesthetics • Positive inotropes • Sympathomimetics
- Hypotension

KEY POINTS

- Blood pressure monitoring is essential in perioperative patients, and recognition and appropriate therapy are critical for successful outcomes in these patients.
- There are numerous mechanisms that a patient will use to try to maintain normal blood pressure and perfusion, but many of the anesthetic agents that are used may inhibit their ability to regulate blood pressure.
- Hypotension during anesthesia can be caused by decreased cardiac output (secondary to decreased heart rate, stroke volume, or both) or decreased systemic vascular resistance, or a combination of both.
- Treatment of hypotension should be directed by identification of the underlying cause of the hypotension.

Blood pressure is a vital parameter to monitor in the perioperative period. Major fluctuations with either hypotension or less commonly hypertension can have serious consequences for the patient. How susceptible the patient is to damage from abnormal blood pressure will be variable depending on if there are any underlying illnesses. As an example, a patient with renal disease will have lost renal autoregulation, a mechanism by which the body maintains normal glomerular filtration rate and renal blood flow over a wide range of blood pressures.[1] Without autoregulation, the kidney will lose blood flow and glomerular filtration rate at blood pressures at which healthy animals would have no deleterious effects. As such, it is vital that each patient be assessed for potential risk factors for blood pressure dysregulation.

The authors have nothing to disclose.
Department of Small Animal Clinical Sciences, Western College Veterinary Medicine, University of Saskatchewan, 52 Campus Drive, Saskatoon, Saskatchewan S7N 5B4, Canada
* Corresponding author.
E-mail address: endovet@juno.com

Vet Clin Small Anim 45 (2015) 965–981
http://dx.doi.org/10.1016/j.cvsm.2015.04.004
0195-5616/15/$ – see front matter © 2015 Elsevier Inc. All rights reserved.

To manage blood pressure, it is necessary to measure blood pressure accurately; unfortunately, this is very challenging. Generally, either direct or indirect methods are used. Direct blood pressures have been considered the gold standard for measurement and are often used in very critical patients. Data have shown however that even direct blood pressures can be discordant in cats[2] and dogs.[3] The discrepancy is great enough that if the criteria for blood pressure device validation were applied in comparing carotid artery blood pressure values to dorsal pedal or femoral artery pressures in dogs, none of the systolic values obtained would be acceptable.[4] Indirect monitors have also been considered inaccurate, although at times this may be because the direct methods used were not reliable or appropriately carried out. There are certainly significant issues with managing blood pressure when the numbers obtained by any method have to be questioned. Nonetheless, blood pressure monitoring is vital, although at times it is important to realize that trends are the predominant thing being monitored because absolute numbers often are elusive. It is also important that blood pressure monitoring in the perioperative period be consistent. Given the variability of the numbers generated by various methodologies, it is advisable to use the same method in a patient being monitored to be able to more readily identify trends. It is also advisable that whatever technique is used is a technique the operator is experienced with to be able to troubleshoot any problems that occur.

BLOOD PRESSURE CONTROL

Arterial blood pressure is controlled by many mechanisms, all of which interact to provide optimal tissue perfusion under different circumstances. These mechanisms can be classified according to the time period in which they respond to a situation and act to perform a correction.

Ultra-Short-Acting Blood Pressure Control Systems

Autoregulation systems can adapt to changes produced by anesthetic agents, although these mechanisms may still be affected by certain drugs. Metabolic nitric oxide results in vasodilation increasing blood flow to the tissue-enhancing removal of waste products and increasing delivery of oxygen and nutrients. A continual supply of nitric oxide is required because it has a very short lifespan (nanoseconds).

Individual organs, such as the brain and kidney, can use a similar and more refined system of organ autoregulation, which ensures a steady blood flow to the whole tissue during periods of hypotension. Other organ systems that do not have mechanisms of autoregulation, such as the gastrointestinal tract, rapidly become debilitated during prolonged periods of hypotension.

Short-Acting Blood Pressure Control Systems

The control of blood pressure provided by the autonomic nervous system (ANS) is most relevant to the period of anesthesia. The response time for the ANS to accommodate tissue perfusion requirements is on the order of seconds to minutes, and many changes produced by the ANS can be observed with the aid of monitoring equipment and techniques. The physiology and management of the ANS in critically ill animals have been extensively reviewed elsewhere.[5]

Baroreceptors within the aortic arch and the carotid sinus detect the stretch produced by pressure from blood flow. An increasing degree of stretch increases the neural input to the vasomotor center via the glossopharyngeal nerve (carotid sinus baroreceptors) and vagus nerve (aortic arch baroreceptors). The efferent arm of this reflex is the vagus nerve. Increased mean arterial pressure (MAP) causes an increase in vagal tone, which slows cardiac pacemaker activity. A decrease in baroreceptor firing reduces vagal tone and allows the heart rate (HR) to increase. The cardiac accelerator nerves (lower cervical and upper thoracic spinal nerves) also increase HR in times of SNS activation. In this way, cardiac output (CO) can be readily modified through neural input/output in a matter of seconds. Baroreceptors are also present in other areas of the body, such as the venae cavae, pulmonary veins, atria, ventricles, and pericardium. Right atrial stretch receptors respond to an increased venous return by increasing HR; this reflex is known as the Bainbridge reflex.[6]

Aortic arch and carotid body chemoreceptors respond to both decreasing partial pressure of oxygen and increasing partial pressure of carbon dioxide, and these changes will increase ventilation, increase sympathetic nervous system (SNS) tone, and improve tissue perfusion.

Long-Acting Control Systems

The long-acting renin–angiotensin–aldosterone system and atrial natriuretic peptide secretion control systems are important for patient management during anesthesia, but their slow time course of action over days makes them less amenable to manipulation during the anesthetic period. Antidiuretic hormone (ADH) is normally secreted in minute amounts, but if there is a severe decrease of circulating volume, ADH is secreted in high amounts to produce vasoconstriction. However, in these circumstances, ADH stores usually exhaust after about an hour, and administration of exogenous vasopressin is occasionally required in debilitated animals. Vasopressin is the only drug used during anesthesia and recovery because its onset of action is rapid, and it can increase blood pressure when catecholamines have failed.[7]

Causes of Hypotension During Anesthesia

Most anesthetic drugs will cause dose-dependent cardiopulmonary depression, affecting vasomotor tone or CO or both. Animals should have enough cardiovascular reserve to cope with the changes in hemodynamics during anesthesia. Preanesthetic stabilization and replacement of lost vascular volume are vital. It is helpful to classify hypotension as mild (MAP 45–60 mm Hg) or severe (MAP <35–45 mm Hg) and assess the speed at which hypotension occurs.

Mild hypotension usually follows a trend and is commonly observed in even healthy anesthetized animals as a result of the combined effects of reduced CO and vasodilation. Inhalant agents such as isoflurane produce vasodilation, while dexmedetomidine may produce bradycardia and reduce cardiac contractility. The overall state of the cardiovascular system requires assessment as well as anesthetic depth and any changes within the respiratory system. If hypotension is present in conjunction with bradycardia, it may be reasonable to try using an anticholinergic drug to reduce vagal tone and improve CO. Reducing the inspired isoflurane level may help restore blood pressure without resorting to extra fluid therapy or sympathomimetics. Isoflurane concentration may be reduced by providing analgesia from other drugs, such as opioid, ketamine, and even α-2 agonist intravenous infusions, which do not have as much effect on hemodynamics.[8]

Severe hypotension, especially if sudden in onset, requires more aggressive diagnosis and correction. Causes of sudden decrease in blood pressure can include a sudden reduction in HR or cardiac contractility from cardiac arrhythmias, hypoxemia, electrolyte or pH disturbances, vasovagal or vagovagal reflexes; massive vasodilation from hypersensitivity reactions, or inflammatory mediator release; sudden reduction in venous return from blood loss, surgical/physical disruption of venous return, pulmonary thromboembolism, tension pneumothorax, and accidental closed breathing system exhaust valve.

Animals affected by disease can have additional factors to consider if hypotension occurs. Chronically hypertensive patients can become unstable during anesthesia and can alternate between periods of profound hypotension and hypertension. Other factors that may be responsible for decreased CO during this period include the presence of myocardial hypoxia, depletion of endogenous catecholamines, metabolic imbalances such as severe acidosis, and electrolyte imbalances. Adequate cortisol concentrations are required for proper adrenoceptor function, and low concentrations may reduce the effectiveness of treatment with catecholamines.

Indirect Indicators of Hypotension

Poor tissue perfusion and reduced oxygen delivery can cause the following:

- Low urine production (<1.0 mL/kg/h)
- Increased blood lactate concentration (>2.0 mmol/L)
- Decreased mixed venous Po_2 (<35 mm Hg) or venous oxygen hemoglobin saturation (<60% sat)
- Slow recovery from anesthesia.

Organ damage is prevented in part during anesthesia through the use of high inspired levels of oxygen, decreased metabolic demand under anesthesia, and the vasodilatory nature of isoflurane and sevoflurane. However, significant hypotension can lead to renal failure and reduced hepatic function, hypoxemia, abnormalities of the central nervous system (including blindness), and cardiac arrest.

CONDITIONS THAT MAY ALSO CAUSE HYPOTENSION
Hypoxemia

Hypoxemia is a stressor, and there is usually stimulation of the SNS. Mild hypoxemia (oxygen hemoglobin saturation of 80%–90%) increases ventilation and CO. The effectiveness of these maneuvers will depend on the cause of hypoxemia. Moderate hypoxemia (oxygen hemoglobin saturation of 60%–80%) causes depletion of energy substrates and some decompensation follows. Peripheral vasodilation and hypotension occur as autoregulation increases perfusion to improve delivery of oxygen. CO diminishes as the myocardium becomes hypoxic. Severe hypoxemia (oxygen hemoglobin saturation of <60%) causes a precipitous decrease in blood pressure and HR, and death can follow if there is no intervention.

Hypercapnia

Increased carbon dioxide levels also cause an increase in SNS tone and systolic arterial pressure (SAP), and CO is maintained or increased. Carbon dioxide is a direct smooth muscle relaxant and diastolic arterial pressure (DAP) tends to decrease from vasodilation. Pulse pressure will widen and peripheral pulses will take on a bounding feel. The vasodilation results in a deep red coloration of mucous membranes. Most anesthetized animals have CO_2 levels of around 50 to 55 mm Hg. The mild increase in SNS tone might be considered an advantage to support blood pressure, but levels greater than 60 to 65 mm Hg should be avoided. In dogs, carbon dioxide levels greater than 70 to 80 mm Hg can cause SAP and HR to increase to around 200 mm Hg and greater than 200 beats/min, respectively. The cause of hypercapnia should be corrected, and these high levels are often a result of a technical failure such as endobronchial intubation or breathing system malfunction.

Intermittent Positive Pressure Ventilation

Intermittent positive pressure ventilation and the use of positive end-expiratory pressure valves can decrease venous return and therefore CO. If continual lung ventilation is used, a shorter inspiratory phase and decreased peak inspiratory pressure can reduce the effect on venous return, but hypoventilation should be avoided.[9]

Local Anesthetics Used for Spinal or Epidural

The use of local anesthetics, such as lidocaine or bupivacaine, in the epidural space of cats and dogs can interrupt SNS outflow from the thoracolumbar spinal cord. Blocked spinal nerves decrease vasomotor tone, and vasodilation will occur. Conscious healthy dogs have little change in blood pressure when these drugs are administered to the level of the thoracolumbar junction.[10] If dogs are hypovolemic or anesthetized with volatile anesthetics, concurrent fluid therapy and vasopressors, such as dopamine or ephedrine, may be required to maintain blood pressure.[11-13]

Surgical Procedures and Position of Animal

Procedures that involve handling of the great veins can limit venous return to the heart. The hypotension is often temporary and can be linked to surgical manipulations. No treatment is usually required except to use gentle surgical technique. If hypotension continues, increasing the rate of fluid therapy and using ephedrine or dopamine should be considered.

Lowering the caudal part of the body below heart level can reduce venous return and promote hypotension. Fluid therapy and ephedrine can be used if the body position cannot be changed to a horizontal position. Tilting the cranial part of the body below heart level will increase venous return.[14]

Abdominal Distention

Gastric dilatation, gas-filled intestines (including gas used for endoscopy), capnoperitoneum, and ascites can decrease venous return and increase afterload.[15] Aggressive fluid therapy may be required if the animal is also hypovolemic, and reduction of pressure, if possible, should be attempted.

Closed Exhaust Valve on the Anesthetic Breathing System

Closed exhaust valve on the anesthetic breathing system can have serious consequences on venous return by increasing intrathoracic pressure and compressing the thin-walled great veins. Peripheral pulses may not be palpable once breathing system pressure increases to more than 20 cm H_2O. Vigilance is important and warning or safety devices on the anesthetic machine will aid in rapid correction.[16]

Tension Pneumothorax

Severe hypotension can follow the development of a tension pneumothorax and is often complicated by hypoxemia. Immediate thoracocentesis is both diagnostic and therapeutic.[17]

Electrolyte and Acid/Base Imbalances

Hyperkalemia, hypocalcemia, and acidosis will decrease myocardial contractility and blood pressure. These problems need to be corrected before blood pressure can be restored.

Hypothermia

Bradycardia can occur if the body temperature is decreased.[18,19] Cats can become hypotensive, and blood pressure often responds to rewarming. Aggressive fluid therapy should not be used in a hypothermic cat because fluid overload may occur in the vasoconstricted state.[20]

Pulmonary embolism

Air or a blood clot may be released into the venous circulation.[21,22] The air or clot will interfere with venous return to the left side of the circulation and CO suddenly drops. As perfusion drops, there will be sudden poor-quality sound from a Doppler probe, and a pulse oximeter will either fail to register a signal or display a low oxygen saturation reading. A capnogram will display a sudden decrease in expired CO_2 from the lungs. Treatment involves removing the air from the ventricles using a jugular catheter, or in emergency, intracardiac aspiration.

Hypersensitivity Reaction

Hypersensitivity reactions are rare, but profound hypotension can result through vasodilation.[23] Histamine release can result from rapid intravenous administration of morphine or meperidine. Treatment depends on severity. Antihistamines can be used for mild hypotension, and epinephrine can be used for severe hypotension, especially if bronchoconstriction is also present.

BLOOD PRESSURE SUPPORT
Fluid Therapy

Fluid therapy improves venous return and CO and replaces fluids lost through bleeding from surgical sites and evaporation of water from exposed body cavities and the lungs. Fluid therapy should be considered an important step in the prevention and treatment of hypotension. Fluid therapy requirements during anesthesia have been reviewed elsewhere, and current recommendations are to provide isotonic replacement crystalloids at a rate of 2 to 3 mL/kg/h for cats and 2 to 6 mL/kg/h for dogs and adjust the rate as required.[24]

In hypotensive animals, an intravenous fluid bolus of 10 mL/kg can be administered over a period of 15 minutes and repeated if necessary until there is improvement in arterial blood pressure or decrease in HR. Overzealous administration of fluids should be avoided; otherwise, interstitial and tissue edema can increase the perfusion distance for oxygen to reach cells. Colloids can be given at a rate of 2.5 to 5 mL/kg over a period of 10 to 15 minutes, and the response can be assessed. Most colloids should not be given at doses of greater than 20 mL/kg in a 24-hour period to avoid hemodilution and coagulopathy.[25]

Anticholinergics

Anticholinergic agents can reverse a vagally mediated bradycardia by blocking M_2 muscarinic receptors at the postganglionic synaptic junctions in areas of the heart innervated by the vagus nerve. During periods of bradycardia, there is more time for diastolic run-off to occur, reducing DAP and MAP while SAP can still be within an acceptable range. A normal SAP with a low MAP and DAP can indicate the HR is physiologically too low.

Occasionally, as a result of removing vagal influence, anticholinergic agents can cause the HR to increase rapidly, leading to tachycardia. Tachycardia usually occurs if the underlying SNS tone is high because of, for example, concurrent hypercapnia or another cause of stress. The anticholinergic drug can unmask the high SNS tone. In such situations, the HR will usually decrease over the following period of approximately 15 minutes.

Atropine
Atropine is a lipophilic molecule (tropane plant alkaloid) and is capable of crossing the blood–brain barrier and placenta. It has a rapid onset of action, and its duration of action is approximately 20 to 40 minutes. It is contraindicated in patients in which ocular drainage is compromised by mydriasis; this can exacerbate glaucoma. Atropine should be used for life-threatening emergencies because it has a more rapid onset of action compared with glycopyrrolate.

- Bolus dose: 0.02 to 0.04 mg/kg intravenously, intramuscularly, subcutaneously.

Glycopyrrolate
Glycopyrrolate may produce a more controlled increase in HR and have a longer onset time compared with atropine. It is a large, ionized molecule (synthetic quaternary amine) and does not cross the blood–brain barrier or the placenta. Its uptake from intramuscular and especially subcutaneous sites is slow. The lower end of the dose range provided can be used to treat bradycardia in large dogs, but it is recommended to use the higher dose rate for smaller dogs and cats to achieve reliable increase in HR.[26] After administration of glycopyrrolate, it can take several minutes for any action to become obvious. It is a powerful antisialogogue and dries up salivary and bronchial secretions. These drying effects can last 2 to 4 hours, whereas the effects on HR may last 1 to 2 hours.

- Bolus dose: 0.005 to 0.01 mg/kg intravenously, intramuscularly, subcutaneously.

Sympathomimetics

Sympathomimetics (inotropes and vasopressors) should always complement fluid therapy and rarely be used as a replacement. The half-lives of catecholamines are short (2–3 minutes); therefore, most catecholamines are administered as a constant rate intravenous infusion. If necessary, bolus doses can be administered, but this should be done with care and with the ability to monitor the response.

Vasopressors are not usually used for mild hypotension, although there is an increasing trend to use these drugs with the increased use of vasodilatory inhalant anesthetic agents such as isoflurane and sevoflurane. The increased arterial blood pressure produced by these drugs may not necessarily suggest there is increased tissue perfusion and oxygen delivery. In fact, it may decrease in the splanchnic region and in skin; for this reason, vasopressors should be used for as short a period as possible. Potent vasopressors are more often used in animals with severe, life-threatening hypotension or in redistributive shock.[27]

Inotropes are especially effective in treating hypotension when combined with intravenous fluid therapy. Many anesthetic agents will cause a degree of myocardial depression, and inotropes are useful to improve myocardial contractility.[28,29]

Mixed inotropes and vasopressors
Drugs with a mixed action may be used during the perianesthetic period. These drugs provide an increase in inotropy and occasionally chronotropy alongside some pressor action. The final result often depends on the dose rate used.

Dopamine Dopamine is the chemical precursor to norepinephrine and epinephrine. Dopaminergic effects are prominent at low infusion rates; β-1-inotropic and chronotropic effects are produced at midrange infusion rates, and α-1-receptor stimulation produces vasoconstriction at high infusion rates. As a result, dopamine can be used as either an inotrope or a vasopressor, depending on the infusion rate. Cardiac arrhythmias may be observed with dopamine, as a result of stimulation of endogenous release of norepinephrine within the heart and its action on α-1 receptors.

Using dopamine in dogs (3–10 µg/kg/min) has been found to increase renal blood flow, which may be due to stimulation of dopamine-1 receptors in the renal vasculature causing vasodilatation, or an increase in CO.[28,30] High-dose dopamine can induce diuresis in cats, but the effect may not be mediated through dopamine receptors.[30] Low-dose dopamine was found to be ineffective.[31] Acepromazine reduces the vasopressor effect of dopamine in dogs anesthetized with isoflurane.[32]

Dopamine administered at a midrange infusion rate increases CO, systemic vascular resistance (SVR), MAP, and HR.

- Low-infusion rate (dopaminergic): 2 to 5 µg/kg/min.
- Midrange infusion rate (β-1): 5 to 10 µg/kg/min.
- High-infusion rate (α-1): 10 to 15 µg/kg/min.

Ephedrine Ephedrine stimulates the release of endogenous norepinephrine, which produces its sympathomimetic action at both α- and β-adrenoceptors. Ephedrine is the ideal drug for the correction of mild hypotension, where aggressive treatment is not necessary.[33] As norepinephrine stores are used, the effect of subsequent ephedrine boluses diminishes, although ephedrine also has some direct action on adrenoceptors. Ephedrine decreases renal and splanchnic perfusion, but the reduction in renal perfusion is not as great as that produced by directly acting α-1-adrenergic agonists. Ephedrine increases MAP, HR, and CO. It has a particularly useful vasoconstrictor action on the great veins and increases venous return.

It is possible, although not necessary, to give ephedrine as an infusion.[34]

- Bolus dose: 0.02 to 0.05 mg/kg intravenously, intramuscularly.
- Infusion rate: 1 to 5 µg/kg/min.

Norepinephrine Norepinephrine stimulates β-1 receptors, but not β-2 receptors, and increases inotropy and CO. Its effect on α-1 receptors is powerful and dose dependent. Norepinephrine increases SVR, thus limiting any effective increase in CO when given at higher infusion rates. Perfusion of the liver, kidneys, muscles, and skin is reduced, and therefore, the drug should be administered for as short a time as possible. However, its powerful vasoconstrictive effects are useful in patients with redistributive shock.[27]

- Infusion rate: 0.1 to 1.0 µg/kg/min.

Epinephrine Epinephrine is a powerful inotrope, chronotrope, and vasopressor. It is usually reserved for life-threatening situations, such as severe hypotension, anaphylactic shock, or cardiac arrest. The overall effects are dose dependent, with higher doses stimulating more α receptors in the vascular system. β-1 stimulation increases HR and CO. Both DAP and MAP may remain constant or decrease because of β-2-mediated vasodilation within skeletal muscle. Because MAP does not change, the baroreceptor reflex arc is not triggered and bradycardia does not usually occur.[4]

- Bolus dose: 0.01 to 0.1 mg/kg intravenously, intramuscularly.
- Infusion rate: 0.01 to 0.03 µg/kg/min.

Inotropes

For immediate improvement in myocardial contractility, dobutamine is commonly used, although dopamine can be used at the appropriate infusion rate.

Dobutamine Dobutamine is a synthetic catecholamine and produces a dose-dependent increase in CO through β-1-receptor stimulation. SVR does not usually change or may decrease, and coronary artery dilation occurs. There is little risk of cardiac arrhythmias with dobutamine because endogenous norepinephrine is not released. Occasionally, dobutamine causes an increase in HR without an appreciable increase in MAP.[27,35] Animals responding to dobutamine with tachycardia may be sensitive to the drug effects and require lower infusion rates, or more fluid therapy to increase venous return.

- Infusion rate: 2 to 10 μg/kg/min.

Vasopressors

Vasopressors can increase arterial blood pressure and SVR.[27,36] They rarely will increase and most often will reduce CO, especially at high doses. They should be given for short periods and should be removed as soon as possible. Excessively high arterial pressure can force fluids out of the circulation into the extracellular fluid compartment and exacerbate hypovolemic states. It can then be difficult to wean these patients from vasopressor therapy, and they become vasopressor-dependent; ultimately this can be detrimental. In this situation, increasing fluid therapy and reducing the α-1-agonist infusion is usually required. Blood pressure measurement is important to ensure arterial pressure is not too high.

Phenylephrine Phenylephrine stimulates α-1 receptors and decreases splanchnic perfusion while increasing SVR. It is useful for treating hypotension mediated through vasodilation and is similar to norepinephrine. Decreased CO can occur through increased afterload (increased MAP and SVR), resulting in a reflex bradycardia.

- Bolus dose: 0.002 to 0.02 mg/kg intravenously.
- Infusion rate: 1 to 3 μg/kg/min.

Vasopressin

Vasopressin stimulates dedicated vasopressin receptors and thus can have an effect even when treatment with catecholamines fails.[27,37] The powerful vasoconstrictive effects of vasopressin can decrease the perfusion of the extremities and the viscera; therefore, vasopressin should be used at the lowest effective infusion rate and for as short a period as possible. Vasopressin can be used alongside dobutamine in extremely debilitated patients.

- Bolus dose: 0.2 to 0.6 IU/kg.
- Infusion rate: 0.002 to 0.006 IU/kg/min.

CARDIOVASCULAR ACTIONS OF DRUGS USED FOR PREANESTHETIC MEDICATION
Acepromazine

Acepromazine can decrease systemic arterial pressure mainly through peripheral vascular α-1-receptor blockade, depression of the vasomotor center, and the myocardium. Administration of 0.11 mg/kg acepromazine intravenously in dogs can decrease MAP by approximately 19% to about 80 mm Hg.[38] Acepromazine has been found to be somewhat protective of renal perfusion despite producing a lower MAP in anesthetized dogs.[39]

Benzodiazepines

This drug may cause excitement in some patients and is not usually given alone. There are, however, no real cardiovascular effects in dogs when benzodiazepines are used at clinical doses.

α-2 Adrenergic Agonists

α-2 agonists have dramatic effects on the cardiovascular system and the reversal agent (eg, yohimbine, tolazoline, or atipamezole) should be available.[40] If bradycardia is considered to be problematic with an increased SVR, the entire dose of reversal or a portion of it can be administered. It is not well understood how low the HR should become before there are problems of tissue perfusion, but a rough guide is to treat any HR that is less than half of the animal's awake and resting value. If there is concurrent hypotension from use of isoflurane, it might be appropriate to use an anticholinergic to avoid losing some beneficial effects of the α-2 agonist. Giving an anticholinergic to treat bradycardia when there is increased SVR present may cause reduced myocardial perfusion and is not recommended.

Xylazine

In dogs, intravenous xylazine causes decreased HR, myocardial contractility, and CO, while blood pressure (MAP around 130 mm Hg), central venous pressure, and SVR are increased. Decreased CO is mainly due to profound bradycardia, and a 235% increase in SVR.[41] The addition of atropine to xylazine can intensify the increase in blood pressure, and MAP can reach 220 mm Hg.[42] Intramuscular administration of xylazine produces similar effects in dogs.[43]

Medetomidine and dexmedetomidine

Medetomidine is a more potent α-2 agonist with less α-1 receptor activity compared with xylazine.[40] Despite this, medetomidine and dexmedetomidine produce similar cardiovascular changes as xylazine. In dogs, administration of 10 μg/kg medetomidine intravenously produces an increased MAP between 140 and 160 mm Hg, which decreases to 90 to 110 mm Hg over the following hour with an accompanying bradycardia.[44] Cats also have a hypertensive response and bradycardia similar to dogs.[45] There does not seem to be as large a decrease in blood pressure from the centrally induced reduction in SNS tone in dogs and cats sedated with medetomidine or dexmedetomidine, compared with changes observed with xylazine.[40] Subsequent anesthesia with isoflurane and sevoflurane will reduce arterial blood pressure, although bradycardia may continue.

OPIOIDS
Morphine

Morphine administration produces a decrease in HR and an initial mild increase in CO and MAP, followed by a reduction in MAP.[46] The initial pressor response is mediated peripherally and the later hemodynamic effects are centrally mediated. Morphine should be administered slowly intravenously because of the potential for histamine release.[47]

Meperidine (Pethidine)

In conscious dogs, administration of 6 mg/kg slow intravenously was found to decrease mesenteric blood flow, SVR, and MAP and to increase HR and renal blood flow. CO increased and then decreased compared with baseline values.[48] Meperidine causes histamine release, and it has been reported to cause a profound decrease in SAP to 20 mm Hg (Doppler technique) in a dog.[49] Therefore, it is not advisable to administer meperidine by this route.

Methadone, Hydromorphone, Oxymorphone

Histamine is minimally released by these opioids, and systolic blood pressure is maintained. Five minutes after intravenous administration of oxymorphone (0.1 mg/kg) in dogs does not appreciably change MAP. After 0.4 mg/kg intravenously, MAP and SVR increase, HR decreases, and CO transiently decreases.[50] In dogs, oxymorphone intravenously followed by midazolam intravenously produces hemodynamically stable conditions with a slight decrease in MAP.[51]

Butorphanol and Buprenorphine

In halothane-anesthetized dogs, butorphanol (0.2 mg/kg intravenously) will decrease MAP and HR.[52] In awake dogs, buprenorphine administered at a dose of 16 μg/kg intravenously produces mild decreases in MAP, CO, and HR.[53]

INDUCTION OF ANESTHESIA

The hemodynamic changes that occur during induction of anesthesia can result in hypotension. Clinical doses of alfaxalone, propofol, or thiopental for induction of anesthesia depress the vasomotor center, causing global vasodilation. The drugs may also depress myocardial contractility to some degree and reduce CO. The ability of compensatory mechanisms to restore blood pressure is also temporarily reduced. The HR often increases via activation of the baroreceptor reflex arc and can restore blood pressure. Propofol, however, resets the baroreceptor threshold, so there is reduced ability to increase HR compared with the increases in HR observed with alfaxalone and thiopental. This reduced ability to compensate for hypotension can make propofol a less favorable choice for induction of anesthesia in hypovolemic animals.

The degree of hypotension produced by injectable anesthetic agents may be offset by giving the drug slowly over a period of 60 seconds and by using coinduction techniques with benzodiazepines.[54] Intubation of the trachea can stimulate the SNS and increase HR and arterial blood pressure. If this response is undesirable, anesthetic depth should be ensured at surgical plane, or topical lidocaine can be used on the laryngeal mucosa before intubation. In dogs, injection of intravenous lidocaine was not found to suppress this SNS response.[55]

INJECTABLE ANESTHETIC DRUGS
Thiopental

Thiopental produces the previously described hemodynamic effects when used for induction of anesthesia. In healthy dogs, induction doses of thiopental maintained MAP.[56] Thiopental produces an increase in HR and little myocardial depression, but contractility is reduced at higher doses. Thiopental has the potential to be arrhythmogenic and can cause ventricular premature contractions. In cats with meperidine/acepromazine/atropine given for preanesthetic medication, thiopental did not change HR, SVR, or MAP. Decreased cardiac index and stroke volume were attributed to the premedication drugs.[57] In hypovolemic dogs, induction doses of thiopental caused a profound decrease in MAP, but an increase in HR returned MAP to around 76 mm Hg.[58]

Propofol

Propofol causes decreased blood pressure by reducing vasomotor tone as described earlier, but seems to have more direct dilatory effect on the great veins.[59] The HR does not seem to increase sufficiently to compensate for hypotension. In healthy acepromazine/hydromorphone premedicated dogs, MAP decreased to 60 to 70 mm Hg after induction.[60] In hypovolemic dogs, propofol decreased MAP to around 31 mm Hg, although MAP returned to around 50 mm Hg 3 minutes after induction.[61] Propofol should be given slowly and at reduced doses in hypovolemic or septicemic animals. In dogs given an intravenous infusion of propofol (0.4 mg/kg/min), MAP remained around 80 to 90 mm Hg; therefore, infusions for maintenance of anesthesia can provide good hemodynamic stability.[60]

Alfaxalone

The effects of clinical doses of alfaxalone on hemodynamics seem to be minimal.[62] In dogs, SAP changed from approximately 140 to 125 mm Hg in the 10-minute period following injection. CO remained stable through an increase in HR. In cats, although a dose-dependent cardiopulmonary depression was observed, MAP remained around 100 to 110 mm Hg, and HR and CO decreased slightly after clinical doses of alfaxalone.[63] An intravenous infusion of alfaxalone produces stable hemodynamic effects in premedicated dogs.[60]

Etomidate

Etomidate tends to decrease SVR with little effect on myocardial function, and it did not change hemodynamics in hypovolemic dogs.[64] However, etomidate should not be used in septicemic or immunosuppressed animals because it suppresses the adrenocortical axis.[65]

Ketamine and Benzodiazepine Combinations

Ketamine alone increases MAP through central stimulation of the SNS, but addition of a benzodiazepine will blunt this response.[66,67] In healthy dogs, MAP remains around 110 to 120 mm Hg a few minutes after administration. In hypovolemic dogs, ketamine/diazepam produced the least disruption in hemodynamics compared with thiopental and propofol and is probably the induction agent of choice in hypovolemic or septicemic animals.[54] However, there should still be some attempt to stabilize the patient with adequate fluid therapy before anesthesia is induced.

Tiletamine/Zolazepam Combination

In dogs and cats, Telazol intravenously causes a dose-dependent depression of MAP to between 60 and 80 mm Hg 5 minutes following induction due to decreased SVR and CO.[68]

INHALATIONAL ANESTHETIC DRUGS
Isoflurane and Sevoflurane

The SVR is reduced with isoflurane and sevoflurane through a direct vasodilatory action on the vasculature smooth muscle. These drugs also reduce myocardial contractility. Mechanisms include the following:

- Decreased availability of calcium ions for muscle contraction
- Inhibition of central sympathetic outflow
- Decreased formation of cyclic AMP
- Peripheral autonomic ganglion blockade
- Attenuated carotid body reflex activity

In dogs, the cardiopulmonary effects of sevoflurane and isoflurane are similar with dose-dependent cardiopulmonary effects.[69] In cats breathing sevoflurane, a dose-dependent decrease in myocardial contractility and decrease in SAP to around 80 to 90 mm Hg was observed, with little change in HR, SVR, and central venous pressure.[70]

Box 1
Cause of hypotension in the perioperative patient

Problems involving CO

Reduced stroke volume

- Reduced venous return and ventricular filling (treatment: intravenous fluids, α-1 agonists)
- Reduced cardiac contractility (treatment: β-1 agonists)

Heart rate

- Bradycardia (treatment: anticholinergics, β-1 agonists)
- HRs at the low end of normal do not usually affect CO
- Extreme tachycardia (establish the cause and treat accordingly)

Problems involving SVR

- Excessive vasodilation (treatment: intravenous fluids, α-1 agonists, vasopressin).

Nitrous Oxide

Nitrous oxide administered alone maintains blood pressure through SNS stimulation, but it has direct myocardial depressant actions. The addition of nitrous oxide to isoflurane and sevoflurane can improve blood pressure through stimulation of the SNS, and by providing enough analgesia to allow a reduction in inspired volatile agent. In dogs, this stimulatory action seems more pronounced with the use of sevoflurane, compared with isoflurane.[71]

SUMMARY

Hypotension can develop in patients in the perioperative period because of several factors. Identification of the primary problem (decreased CO vs decreased SVR) is essential in deciding on the best treatment option for each patient. **Box 1** can help in the diagnosis and treatment of hypotension. Early recognition and appropriate treatment are essential for optimizing outcome in the perioperative patient.

REFERENCES

1. Brown SA, Finco DR, Navar LG. Impaired renal autoregulatory ability in dogs with reduced renal mass. J Am Soc Nephrol 1995;5:1768–74.
2. Parker K, Carr A, Duke Novakovski T. Not all arteries are created equal: comparison of pressures within the aortic root and the dorsal pedal artery in cats. J Vet Intern Med 2012;26:717.
3. Monteiro AR, Campagnol D, Bajotto GC, et al. Effects of 8 hemodynamic conditions on direct blood pressure values obtained simultaneously from the carotid, femoral and dorsal pedal arteries in dogs. J Vet Cardiol 2013;15:263–70.
4. Brown S, Atkins C, Bagley R, et al. Guidelines for the identification, evaluation and management of systemic hypertension in dogs and cats. J Vet Intern Med 2007; 21:542–8.
5. Long KM, Kirby R. An update on cardiovascular adrenergic receptor physiology and potential pharmacological applications in veterinary medicine. J Vet Emerg Crit Care 2008;18:2–25.
6. Crystal GJ, Ramez Salem M. The Bainbridge and the "reverse" Bainbridge reflexes: history, physiology, and clinical relevance. Anesth Analg 2012;114:520–32.

7. Russell JA. Vasopressin in vasodilatory and septic shock. Curr Opin Crit Care 2007;13:383–91.
8. Duke T. Partial intravenous anesthesia in cats and dogs. Can Vet J 2013;54: 276–82.
9. Hedenstierna G. Pulmonary perfusion during anesthesia and mechanical ventilation. Minerva Anestesiol 2005;71:319–24.
10. Duke T, Caulkett NA, Ball SD, et al. Comparative analgesic and cardiopulmonary effects of bupivacaine and ropivacaine in the epidural space of the conscious dog. Vet Anaesth Analg 2000;27:13–21.
11. Greitz T, Andreen M, Irestedt L. Effects of ephedrine on haemodynamics and oxygen consumption in the dog during high epidural block with special reference to the splanchnic region. Acta Anaesthesiol Scand 1984;28:557–62.
12. Holte K, Foss NB, Svensén C, et al. Epidural anesthesia, hypotension, and changes in intravascular volume. Anesthesiology 2004;100:281–6.
13. Raner C, Biber B, Lundberg J, et al. Cardiovascular depression by isoflurane and concomitant thoracic epidural anesthesia is reversed by dopamine. Acta Anaesthesiol Scand 1994;38:136–43.
14. Avesthey P, Wood EH. Intrathoracic and venous pressure relationships during responses to changes in body position. J Appl Physiol 1974;37:166–75.
15. Diamont M, Benumof JL, Saidman LJ. Hemodynamics of increased intra-abdominal pressure. Anesthesiology 1978;48:22–7.
16. McMurphy R, Hodgson D, Cribb PH. Modification of a nonrebreathing circuit adapter to prevent barotrauma in anesthetized patients. Vet Surg 1995;24: 352–5.
17. Pawloski DR, Broaddus KD. Pneumothorax: a review. J Am Anim Hosp Assoc 2010;46:385–97.
18. Pereira NJ. ECG of the month. J Am Vet Med Assoc 2014;244:1384–6.
19. Wood T, Thorensen M. Physiological responses to hypothermia. Semin Fetal Neonatal Med 2015;20:87–96.
20. Armitage-Chan EA, O'Toole T, Chan DL. Management of prolonged food deprivation, hypothermia, and refeeding syndrome in a cat. Vet Emerg Crit Care 2006;16: S34–41.
21. Goggs R, Benigni L, Fuentes VL, et al. Pulmonary thromboembolism. J Vet Emerg Crit Care 2009;19:30–52.
22. Wilkins RE, Unverdorben M. Accidental intravenous infusion of air. J Infus Nurs 2012;35:404–8.
23. Schmuel DL, Cortes Y. Anaphylaxis in dogs and cats. J Vet Emerg Crit Care 2013; 23:377–94.
24. Davis H, Jensen T, Johnson A, et al. 2013 AAHA/AAFP fluid therapy guidelines for dogs and cats. J Am Anim Hosp Assoc 2013;49:149–59.
25. Cazolli D, Prittie J. The crystalloid-colloid debate: consequences of resuscitation fluid selection in veterinary critical care. J Vet Emerg Crit Care 2015;25: 6–19.
26. Dyson DH, James-Davies R. Dose effect and benefits of glycopyrrolate in the treatment of bradycardia in anesthetized dogs. Can Vet J 1999;40:327–31.
27. Silverstein D, Santoro Beer KA. Controversies regarding choice of vasopressor therapy for management of septic shock in animals. J Vet Emerg Crit Care 2015;25:48–54.
28. Pascoe P, Ilkiw JE, Pypendop PH. Effects of increasing infusion rates of dopamine, dobutamine, epinephrine, and phenylephrine in healthy anesthetized cats. Am J Vet Res 2006;67:1491–9.

29. Rosati M, Dyson DH, Sinclair MD, et al. Response of hypotensive dogs to dopamine hydrochloride and dobutamine hydrochloride during deep isoflurane anesthesia. Am J Vet Res 2007;68:483–94.
30. Sigrist NE. Use of dopamine in acute renal failure. J Vet Emerg Crit Care 2007;17:117–26.
31. Wohl JS, Schwartz DD, Flournoy S, et al. Renal hemodynamic and diuretic effects of low-dose dopamine in anesthetized cats. J Vet Emerg Crit Car 2007;17:45–52.
32. Monteiro ER, Texeira Neto FJ, Castro VB, et al. Effects of acepromazine on the cardiovascular actions of dopamine in anesthetized dogs. Vet Anaesth Analgesia 2007;34:312–21.
33. Chen HC, Sinclair MD, Dyson DH. Use of ephedrine and dopamine in dogs for the management of hypotension in routine clinical cases under isoflurane anesthesia. Vet Anaesth Analgesia 2007;34:301–11.
34. Sinclair MD, Dyson D. The impact of acepromazine on the efficacy of crystalloid, dextran or ephedrine treatment in hypotensive dogs under isoflurane anesthesia. Vet Anaesth Analgesia 2012;39:563–73.
35. Dyson DH, Sinclair MD. Impact of dopamine or dobutamine infusions on cardiovascular variables after rapid blood loss and volume replacement during isoflurane-induced anesthesia in dogs. Am J Vet Res 2006;67:1121–30.
36. Thiele RH, Nemergut EC, Lynch C. The clinical implications of isolated alpha(1) adrenergic stimulation. Anesth Analg 2011;113:297–304.
37. Silverstein DC, Waddell LS, Drobatz KJ, et al. Vasopressin therapy in dogs with dopamine-resistant hypotension and vasodilatory shock. J Vet Emerg Crit Care 2007;17:399–408.
38. Turner DM, Ilkiw JE, Rose RJ, et al. Respiratory and cardiovascular effects of five drugs used as sedatives in the dog. Aust Vet J 1974;50:260–5.
39. Boström I, Nyman G, Kampa N, et al. Effects of acepromazine on renal function in anesthetized dogs. Am J Vet Res 2003;64:590–8.
40. Sinclair MD. A review of the physiological effects of alpha2-agonists related to the clinical use of medetomidine in small animal practice. Can Vet J 2003;44:885–97.
41. Klide AM, Calderwood HW, Soma LR. Cardiopulmonary effects of xylazine in dogs. Am J Vet Res 1975;36:931–5.
42. Hsu WH, Hemborough FB. Effect of xylazine on heart rate and arterial blood pressure in conscious dogs, as influenced by atropine, 4-aminopyridine, doxapram, and yohimbine. J Am Vet Med Assoc 1985;186:153–6.
43. Ilbäck I, Stålhandske T. Cardiovascular effects of xylazine recorded with telemetry in the dog. J Vet Med A Physiol Pathol Clin Med 2003;50:479–83.
44. Pypendop B, Verstegen JP. Hemodynamic effects of medetomidine in the dog: a dose titration study. Vet Surg 1998;27:612–22.
45. Golden AL, Bright JM, Daniel GB, et al. Cardiovascular effects of the alpha2-adrenergic receptor agonist medetomidine in clinically normal cats anesthetized with isoflurane. Am J Vet Res 1998;59:509–13.
46. Maiante AA, Texeira Neto FJ, Beier SL, et al. Comparison of the cardio-respiratory effects of methadone and morphine in conscious dogs. J Vet Pharmacol Ther 2008;32:317–28.
47. Guedes AGP, Papich MG, Rude EP, et al. Comparison of plasma histamine levels after intravenous administration of hydromorphone and morphine in dogs. J Vet Pharmacol Ther 2007;30:516–22.
48. Priano LI, Vatner SF. Generalized cardiovascular and regional hemodynamic effects of meperidine in conscious dogs. Anesth Analg 1981;60:649–54.

49. Dobromylskyj P. Severe hypotension and urticaria following the intravenous administration of pethidine in two dogs. J Vet Anaesth 1992;19:87–8.

50. Haskins SC, Copland VS, Patz JD. The cardiopulmonary effects of oxymorphone in hypovolemic dogs. J Vet Emerg Crit Care 1991;1:32–8.

51. Jacobson JD, McGrath CJ, Smith EP. Cardiorespiratory effects of four opioid-tranquilizer combinations in dogs. Vet Surg 1994;23:299–306.

52. Greene SA, Hartsfield SM, Tyner CL. Cardiovascular effects of butorphanol in halothane-anesthetized dogs. Am J Vet Res 1990;51:1276–9.

53. Martinez EA, Hartsfield SM, Melendez LD, et al. Cardiovascular effects of buprenorphine in anesthetized dogs. Am J Vet Res 1997;58:1280–4.

54. Fayyez S, Kerr CL, Dyson DH, et al. The cardiopulmonary effects of anesthetic induction with isoflurane, ketamine-diazepam or propofol-diazepam in the hypovolemic dog. Vet Anaesth Analgesia 2009;36:110–23.

55. Joliffe CT, Leece EA, Adams V. Effect of intravenous lidocaine on heart rate, systolic arterial blood pressure and cough responses to endotracheal intubation in propofol-anaesthetized dogs. Vet Anaesth Analgesia 2007;34:322–30.

56. Turner DM, Ilkiw JE. Cardiovascular and respiratory effects of three rapidly acting barbiturates in dogs. Am J Vet Res 1990;51:598–604.

57. Dyson DH, Allen DG, Ingwersen W, et al. Evaluation of acepromazine/meperidine/atropine premedication followed by thiopental anesthesia in the cat. Can J Vet Res 1988;52:419–22.

58. Ilkiw JE, Haskins SC, Patz JD. Cardiovascular and respiratory effects of thiopental administration in hypovolemic dogs. Am J Vet Res 1999;52:576–80.

59. Marik PE. Propofol: therapeutic indications and side-effects. Curr Pharm Des 2004;10:3639–49.

60. Ambros A, Duke-Novakovski T, Pasloske K. Comparison of the anesthetic efficacy and cardiopulmonary effects of continuous rate infusions of alfaxalone-2-hydroxypropyl-β-cyclodextrin and propofol in dogs. Am J Vet Res 2008;69:1391–8.

61. Ilkiw JE, Pascoe PJ, Haskins SC, et al. Cardiovascular and respiratory effects of propofol administration in hypovolemic dogs. Am J Vet Res 1992;53:2323–7.

62. Muir WW, Lerche P, Wiese A, et al. Cardiorespiratory and anesthetic effects of clinical and supraclinical doses of alfaxalone in dogs. Vet Anaesth Analgesia 2008;35:451–62.

63. Muir WW, Lerche P, Wiese A, et al. Cardiorespiratory and anesthetic effects of clinical and supraclinical doses of alfaxalone in cats. Vet Anaesth Analgesia 2009;36:42–54.

64. Pascoe PJ, Ilkiw JE, Haskins SC, et al. Cardiopulmonary effects of etomidate in hypovolemic dogs. Am J Vet Res 1992;53:2178–82.

65. Hirschman LJ. The cardiopulmonary and metabolic effects of hypoxia during acute adrenocortical suppression by etomidate in the dog. AANA J 1991;59:282–7.

66. Haskins SC, Farver TB, Patz JD. Ketamine in dogs. Am J Vet Res 1985;46:1855–60.

67. Haskins SC, Farver TB, Patz JD. Cardiovascular changes in dogs given diazepam and diazepam-ketamine. Am J Vet Res 1986;47:795–8.

68. Hellyer P, Muir WW, Hubbell JAE, et al. Cardiorespiratory effects of the intravenous administration of tiletamine-zolazepam to dogs. Vet Surg 1989;18:160–5.

69. Bernard JM, Wouters PF, Doursout MF, et al. Effects of sevoflurane and isoflurane on cardiac and coronary dynamics in chronically instrumented dogs. Anesthesiology 1990;72:659–62.

70. Pypendop BH, Ilkiw JE. Hemodynamic effects of sevoflurane in cats. Am J Vet Res 2004;65:20–5.
71. Duke T, Caulkett NA, Tataryn JM. The effect of nitrous oxide on halothane, isoflurane and sevoflurane requirements in ventilated dogs undergoing ovariohysterectomy. Vet Anaesth Analgesia 2006;33:343–50.

Inadvertent Perianesthetic Hypothermia in Small Animal Patients

Stuart Clark-Price, DVM, MS

KEYWORDS

- Dog • Cat • Anesthesia • Hypothermia • Temperature
- Inadvertent perianesthetic hypothermia

KEY POINTS

- Inadvertent perianesthetic hypothermia is one of the most common complications associated with anesthesia.
- Hypothermia has been associated with may adverse events, including altered pharmacokinetics of anesthetic and analgesic drugs, dysfunction of organ systems, increased patient susceptibility to infection, reduced wound healing, altered coagulation, hypotension, and delayed recovery.
- Heat loss–minimizing techniques should be applied to dogs anesthetized for longer than 20 minutes.
- Heat loss techniques can be passive, active, or metabolic in nature.
- Passive techniques include insulatory materials, such as blankets, to minimize loss of existing body heat.

INTRODUCTION

Core temperature is defined as the temperature at which vital organs are maintained and is the temperature of deep structures of the body as compared with that of peripheral tissues. Core body temperature is maintained at a temperature that optimizes enzyme function and homeostasis and therefore, body temperature is considered a "vital sign."[1] Thermoregulation is the ability of an organism to keep its body temperature within certain boundaries, even when the surrounding temperature is very different. The ability to thermoregulate core body temperature can be disrupted by many conditions, including extreme changes in environment, illness and diseases,

The author has nothing to disclose.
Department of Veterinary Clinical Medicine, College of Veterinary Medicine, University of Illinois, 1008 West Hazelwood Drive, MC-004, Urbana, IL 61802, USA
E-mail address: sccp@illinois.edu

and anesthetic and analgesic drugs. In the operating theater, secondary to environmental and pharmaceutical influences, inadvertent perianesthetic hypothermia (IPH) is likely and an understanding of the physiology and pathophysiology of thermoregulation, effect of drugs, and options for temperature management can enhance patient care.

Physiology of Thermoregulation and the Response to Hypothermia

Core body temperature is one of the most vigorously defended physiologic parameters of the mammalian body and results from a balance of heat production and heat loss. The hypothalamus acts as the major thermoregulatory center or "thermostat" and acts in concert with other minor centers in the skin, abdomen, thorax, spinal cord, and other centers in the brain to define and maintain a set point body temperature.[2,3] Threshold temperatures for activation of heat-generating or cooling physiologic and behavioral changes are set in the posterior hypothalamus. The threshold temperatures for most mammals is a very narrow range of approximately 0.2°C above or below the set point body temperature and in healthy animals thermoregulatory defenses are quite effective.[3] Thermoregulation occurs through a complex mechanism of afferent thermal sensing, central regulation, and efferent responses to changes in environmental and body temperature.[4] Afferent sensing starts with thermally sensitive cells in virtually all tissues within the body. Cold and warm sensitive cells are anatomically and physically distinct from each other.[4] Cold-signaling cells use myelinated A-delta nerve fibers to transmit their impulses to the spinal cord, whereas warm-signaling cells use nonmyelinated C fibers.[3] Myelinated fibers propagate nerve impulses at a greater velocity than nonmyelinated fibers and are better at sending localizing information, and thus cold temperatures may be more rapidly felt and localized to parts of the body. Interestingly, information from pain-sensing neurons also use A-delta and C fibers for signal propagation.[5] Temperature-sensitive receptors for cold and warmth are physiologically distinct and reside in the skin, spinal cord, abdominal viscera, and around the great veins in the upper abdomen and thorax.[6] Within the skin, there is approximately 10 times the number of cold-sensitive receptors compared with warmth-sensitive receptors, suggesting that peripheral detection of cold environmental temperatures has greater physiologic importance.[6] The firing or signaling rate of these temperature-sensitive receptors increases as the surrounding tissue temperature moves away from the established temperature set point. For example, as the skin temperature drops, the cold-sensitive receptors increase the firing rate of nerve impulses that are sent to the spinal cord.

On interfacing with the spinal cord, nerve impulses carrying temperature information travel to higher centers mainly thought spinothalamic tracts in the anterior spinal cord. Various other spinal tracts can convey thermal information to the brain and therefore an organism can elicit some response to changes in temperature even if the spinothalamic tracts are damaged.[4]

The preoptic area in the anterior hypothalamus also contains temperature-sensitive neurons.[6] Heat-sensitive and cold-sensitive neurons respond in much the same manner as those found throughout the body, indicating that core brain temperature is also well regulated. Temperature information from the preoptic area of the anterior hypothalamus is combined with temperature information entering the higher centers from the spinal cord and is directed to the posterior hypothalamus for integration into whole-body temperature regulation. When this information indicates that the body has fallen outside of the temperature set point, appropriate efferent responses are activated to return body temperature to the normal range.

Efferent responses can be divided into body temperature–increasing and body temperature–decreasing activities. Temperature-increasing activities include vasoconstriction and activation of arteriovenous shunts, piloerection, shivering, and metabolic thermogenesis. Temperature-decreasing activities include vasodilation, sweating, panting, and decreased metabolic thermogenesis.

Changes in vascular tone and blood flow, particularly to the skin, are one of the most immediate responses to changes in body temperature. During hypothermia, peripheral cutaneous blood flow is decreased to reduce heat loss through the skin. Blood flow to the skin is functionally divided into 2 types: nutritional, supplied by capillaries; and thermoregulatory, mainly through arteriovenous shunts.[7] These shunts are anatomically distinct from the capillary beds of the skin and do not compromise peripheral tissue metabolic needs. On recognition that body heat conservation is necessary, the arteriovenous shunts are activated to promote centralized blood flow and reduce heat loss through the skin.[4]

Piloerection quite literally means hairs standing on end. For most mammals, including dogs, piloerection is a somewhat effective method of reducing heat loss. Piloerection occurs when musculi arrectores pilorum, the tiny muscles that elevate hair follicles above the skin, contract in response to sympathetic stimulation.[6] This smooth muscle makes a connection from the fibrils to the underlying connective tissue and involuntary contraction occurs in response to catecholamine.[8] The heat retention properties that are a result of piloerection are not related to the properties of the hair, but are because of layers of motionless air that are trapped next to the skin and form an outer layer of insulation. This mechanism allows animals to compensate for a moderately cooling environment without the need to increase metabolism.[8] The effectiveness of piloerection is somewhat dependent on body size. Animals heavier than 5 kg are more likely to benefit from piloerection, whereas it is less effective in smaller animals because of a higher body surface-to-volume ratio.[8,9]

Shivering is an involuntary action of the body whereby skeletal muscle rapidly contracts or twitches. The primary motor center for shivering is located in the posterior hypothalamus near the third ventricle. This area is excited by cold signals from the skin and spinal cord and responds by sending signals to the brain stem and spinal cord, which in turn activates motor neurons.[6] Muscle tone increases and nonrhythmical contractions increase until shivering begins. Shivering can be a quite effective bodily mechanism for hypothermia, as it can increase heat production by fourfold to fivefold.[6] However, heat generation by shivering comes at a tremendous metabolic cost. During shivering, metabolic oxygen consumption increases up to 700%, which may be of critical importance in very sick patients, particularly in a patient with myocardial disease.[10]

In response to hypothermia, the body can manufacture heat as a by-product of metabolism. This can occur directly, as hypothermia can increase metabolism of various cells, including adipose tissue, and indirectly via epinephrine and norepinephrine activation of metabolic pathways.[11] Hypothermia is stressful to the body and results in an increased release of stress-related biochemicals, such as epinephrine and norepinephrine.[6] Part of the metabolic increase of heat production is through the ability of epinephrine and norepinephrine to uncouple oxidative phosphorylation and result in the release of energy in the form of heat instead of production of ATP.[6] The greatest proportion of heat derived from adipose tissue occurs in brown adipose tissue or brown fat; however, protein and carbohydrates also contribute to metabolic heat production.[12] Other metabolic pathways that activate uncoupling proteins also contribute to heat generation, mainly thyrotropin-releasing hormone (TRH). Released by the hypothalamus in response to cooling of the preoptic area, TRH in turn stimulates the anterior pituitary gland to release thyroid-stimulating hormone, which simulates increased release of thyroxine by the thyroid gland.[6] Thyroxine increases cellular metabolism with a resultant increased production of heat as a by-product of this cellular work.

Core Versus Peripheral Temperature and Patterns of Heat Loss

Core body temperature is the temperature of an organism at which it was meant to operate and tends to refer to the temperature of organs and deep structures of the body that are well insulated and tightly regulated. Peripheral body temperature is the temperature that is measured closer to the surface of the body, can vary widely, and is heavily influenced by environmental temperatures. In veterinary medicine, rectal temperature is the most commonly measured temperature. The average rectal temperature measured in healthy dogs is approximately 102°F (38.8°C); however, circadian rhythmicity results in a normal daily range of 100.9° to 102.7°F (38.3°–39.3°C).[13] Core temperature is, on average, approximately 0.72°F (0.4°C) higher than rectal temperature, but can be as much as 2.0°F (1.2°C) higher in healthy dogs at rest.[14] The gold standard for core temperature measurement is in the pulmonary artery; however, this is not the hottest site in the body. Brain tissue has been consistently shown to have the highest tissue temperatures.[15] It is important to have a comprehension of the differences in core versus peripheral temperature so that practitioners can understand how characteristic patterns of heat loss occur in patients during general anesthesia. Core temperature change during anesthesia occurs in 3 phases. During the first hour, there is an initial rapid decline in core temperature, next, over the following 2 hours, core temperature declines in a slower linear fashion, and finally, core temperature stabilizes and remains relatively unchanged (**Fig. 1**).[4] The reason behind this predictable pattern in change in body temperature is a result of the core-to-peripheral temperature gradient and the vasodilation caused by general anesthetics. In awake animals, a temperature gradient of up to 4°C exists between the core and the periphery. This gradient is maintained mainly through peripheral vasoconstriction that keeps body heat in a central pool of blood and thus minimizes the amount of

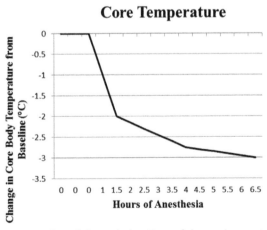

Fig. 1. Graphical representation of the typical pattern of change in core temperature during general anesthesia. There is an initial rapid decline during the first hour, a slower linear decline over the following 2 hours, and then temperature plateaus and remains relatively unchanged.

heat that can be lost through the skin. During anesthesia, the first initial decline in core temperature is a result of peripheral vasodilation and redistribution of body heat. During the second, slower decline, heat loss is directly related to the inhibition of general metabolism and heat production by anesthetic drugs, and results in heat loss in excess of production. The plateau of core temperature after 3 to 4 hours of anesthesia can be seen when a thermal steady state is achieved.

Mechanisms of Heat Loss and Hypothermia

There are 4 main mechanisms of heat loss from the body. These include convection, conduction, radiation, and evaporation (**Table 1**).

- Convection is the loss of body heat to cooler air surrounding the body.
  ○ Example: Operating room environments where room air temperature may be set low for personnel comfort.
- Conduction is the loss of body heat to surfaces that are in contact with the body.
  ○ Example: Stainless steel surgical tables or other hard surfaces that have a temperature lower than the patient's body temperature.
- Radiation is the loss of body heat to structures not in contact with the patient.
  ○ Example: Surgical room walls and equipment within the operating room that have a temperature lower than the patient's body temperature.
- Evaporation is the loss of body heat from evaporating moisture from the body.
  ○ Example: Surgical scrub and alcohol placed directly on the patient and moisture lost from an open body cavity or respiratory secretions.

During general anesthesia, there are many factors that affect the rate of heat loss from each of these 4 mechanisms. These can be divided into environmental factors and patient factors.

Environmental factors include the following:

- Air temperature
- Surrounding object temperature
- Velocity of air movement
- Relative humidity

The difference between the patient's temperature and the temperature of the air or surrounding objects creates a temperature gradient and affects the rate at which heat is lost. The greater the temperature gradient, the greater the rate at which heat is lost from the body. The velocity of air and the relative humidity have an effect on

Table 1		
Mechanisms, physiologic processes, and contributing factors of body heat loss: general anesthesia, environment, and surgical procedures can influence these processes		
Mechanism	**Physiologic Process**	**Example Contributing Factors**
Convection	Transfer of heat from body to surrounding air	Low environmental air temperature, open body cavity
Conduction	Transfer of heat from body to objects in contact	Direct contact with cold, heat-absorbing structures such as stainless steel
Radiation	Transfer of heat from body to objects not in contact	Low environmental temperatures, short or clipped hair coat, open body cavity
Evaporation	Loss of heat from evaporative process	Excessive use of surgical scrub, alcohol, lavage solutions, hair coat soaked with urine or feces

evaporative heat loss. The greater the movement of air and the lower the humidity, the more evaporation occurs and thus more heat is lost.

Patient factors include the following:

- Surface area to body mass ratio
- Physical condition
- Fur type and length
- Disease and injury

As body surface area increases, greater conductive, convective, and radiation heat loss can occur through cutaneous loss. Small and toy-breed dogs are at greater risk because of a higher surface area compared with larger-breed dogs. Physical conditioning of the dog contributes to the rate of heat loss. Muscle can act as heat-generation centers and fat functions as subcutaneous insulation to reduce body heat loss. As can be expected, cachexic and extremely thin animals are at a greater risk for development of hypothermia. Fur type and length play an important role in heat loss in dogs, particularly in arctic breeds such as huskies and malamutes. Longer and thicker fur traps a layer of air next to the body that acts as an insulation to surrounding cooler air and can be particularly effective to reduce convective heat loss. Disease states that reduce metabolic rate or injuries that result in open wounds accelerate heat loss through all 4 mechanisms, as well as negatively impact endogenous heat production.

Anesthetic Effects on Body Temperature

In the perianesthetic period, hypothermia is exacerbated by the anesthetic impairment of the thermoregulatory centers in the hypothalamus.[4] The thermosensitive neurons in the preoptic area of the anterior hypothalamus and the receptors found in the spinal cord, abdominal viscera, and great veins are impaired by most anesthetic and analgesic drugs. The whole-body oxidative metabolism and heat production mechanisms that maintain temperature are silenced.[4] As a result, heat-generating oxidative metabolism is not increased in the face of a falling body temperature, and hypothermia ensues. In addition to the reduction of heat generation, during anesthesia, patients have a reduced ability to conserve previously generated body heat. Most agents used to provide general anesthesia, regional anesthesia, analgesia, or immobilization have been shown to negatively affect thermoregulation.[16,17] Epidural and spinal anesthesia decrease the ability of the thermal centers in the brain to register a decrease in body temperature, as a result, appropriate responses to hypothermia (vasoconstriction, shivering) are blunted. Inhalant anesthetics cause dose-dependent vasodilation and increase the pooling of blood in the peripheral tissues. This increases the surface area of the blood to give up heat to the environment. Opioid analgesic drugs have a direct effect on the central thermostat by lowering the threshold that activates heat-conserving and heat-generating actions of the body, resulting in a colder baseline temperature.

Deleterious Effects of Hypothermia

Hypothermia can have severe detrimental effects to a patient during the perioperative period. In general, hypothermia can alter pharmacokinetics of anesthetic and analgesic drugs, cause dysfunction of organ systems, increase patient susceptibility to infection, reduce wound healing, and alter coagulation.[4,18,19] Enzymatic reactions that are used in metabolism of drugs may be altered, affecting the duration of action of anesthetic drugs. Hypothermia prolongs the action of nondepolarizing paralytic agents.[20] Inhalant anesthetic potency can be influenced by hypothermia. As patient temperature decreases, inhalant anesthetic tissue solubility increases, resulting in increased anesthetic content in body tissues, including the brain, causing increased depth of anesthesia due to a relative anesthetic overdose.[21,22]

Hypothermia can have profound effects on the cardiovascular system through several mechanisms. Alpha receptors show decreased affinity to norepinephrine with subsequent reduced vascular contractility and hypotension.[23–25] Additionally, baroreceptor function decreases as hypothermia ensues, resulting in an inability to increase blood pressure and heart rate in response to changes in volume during anesthesia.[26] Myocardial function can be affected by hypothermia. As body temperature decreases, blood viscosity increases and pH decreases, affecting contracting ability of cardiac myocytes. As the temperature continues to decrease, arrhythmias can develop including ventricular fibrillation.[27,28] The respiratory system is also affected by hypothermia and is clinically characterized by decreased respiratory rate, minute ventilation, and tidal volume, with an increased risk of injury, including pulmonary edema, pneumonia, and acute respiratory distress syndrome.[29,30]

Delayed recovery from anesthesia is a well-known consequence of hypothermia due to decreased central nervous system function; however, hypothermia causes other disturbances in the brain. Cerebral autoregulation is the ability of the brain to regulate blood flow in the face of changes in systemic blood pressure. Hypothermia inhibits the ability of the brain to maintain cerebral blood flow.[31,32]

The immune response and the ability of tissue to heal are also affected by hypothermia. Immunosuppression occurs through inhibition of leukocyte migration, phagocytosis, and decreased synthesis of cytokines.[33] Wound healing is delayed in hypothermia due to decreased inflammatory infiltrates, reduced growth factor production, and less collagen deposition.[34] Hypothermia can even enhance the ability of cancer cells to proliferate.[35]

The clotting system can be profoundly affected by hypothermia. Several processes in the coagulation cascade are impaired by decreased body temperature. Platelet function is affected through decreased aggregation, prothrombin and activated partial thromboplastin clotting times are prolonged, and fibrinolysis can be either accelerated or impaired.[19,30]

INDICATIONS FOR TECHNIQUES TO MINIMIZE HYPOTHERMIA

Using techniques for reducing IPH can improve patient care and reduce side effects associated with hypothermia. The decision on when to use a specific technique depends on the length of the anesthetic event, the procedure, and the patient's condition. In canine patients, techniques to minimize heat loss should be used for anesthetic periods longer than 20 minutes,[36] and may be even more important in feline patients because of their generally smaller size. Additionally, heat loss minimization can be expected to be beneficial in very young, old, or severely ill animals, or those having major surgical or diagnostic procedures. It is also important to remember the IPH carries over into the recovery period. Continued warming therapy after anesthesia and surgery should be part of a standard anesthetic care protocol.

TECHNIQUES AND MECHANISMS OF HEAT CONSERVATION

Techniques for minimizing heat loss in anesthetized patients can be categorized as passive, active, or metabolic. Passive techniques use materials to cover the patient to prevent endogenous heat loss. Passive techniques tend to be minimally effective.[36] Active techniques generate supplemental heat that is externally applied to the patient. Metabolic techniques induce the body to produce increased amounts of endogenous heat through manipulation of metabolism. In veterinary medicine, passive and active techniques are most commonly used.

Passive Techniques

Passive techniques include the use of materials such as cotton towels, newspapers, plastic bubble wrap, and reflective blankets.[36,37] Passive techniques reduce heat loss by counteracting convective and conductive heat loss. They function as an insulator and trap body heat next to the patient. Thus, material that is less permeable to heat, such as plastic or metallic fabrics that reflect heat back to the patient, may be more effective than materials that are more porous. Passive techniques are not nearly as effective as active techniques.

Active Techniques

Active techniques for heat conservation work through application of heat to the patient to reduce the gradient between the body and the environmental temperatures. Electric heating blankets, heat lamps, intravenous fluid warmers, warmed abdominal lavage fluids, circulating warm water pads, resistive polymer electric blankets, and forced warm air blankets are examples of active techniques.[36,38–43] Intravenous fluid warmers appear to have minimal efficacy for combating hypothermia and must be placed on the intravenous fluid line as close to the patient catheter as possible. The use of warmed abdominal lavage solution over room temperature solution in patients undergoing celiotomy can increase the temperature of patients during anesthesia. Lavage solutions should be heated to 43°C and instilled into the abdomen for at least 2 to 6 minutes. Forced warm air blankets seem to be the most efficacious of all the active methods for thermal management in dogs and cats.[4,36,43] Resistive polymer electric blankets have been demonstrated to be both equally and less effective compared with forced warm air blankets.[44,45] Forced warm air blankets can be placed over or under a patient with the direction of the air flow toward the patient. Circulating warm water pads and resistive polymer electric blankets can be placed over or under a patient as well; in addition, because of their flexibility, they can be wrapped around the patient. However, there are drawbacks and limitations to the use of this type of equipment. Blankets and patient coverings can interfere with a surgical field and may have to be positioned on the patient in such a way that it limits the effectiveness. Applying supplemental heating units to the limbs is an effective way to provide heat and maintain access to surgical sites in the abdomen and thorax.[39] Forced warm air units may increase the chance of surgical site infection.[46,47] This is thought to occur through the intake of nonfiltered air or the buildup and emission of microbial contaminants into a surgical field. Equipment that contains ferrous metal is not compatible with certain types of imaging techniques, such as MRI.[48] Additionally, techniques that use blankets or material that covers the patient can interfere with image acquisition and quality of standard radiography, ultrasonography, or computed tomography. Other limitations include cost of purchase, maintenance, replacement of blankets for forced warm air units or circulating warm water pads, inability to easily transport the equipment, and the need for nearby electrical outlets.

Metabolic Techniques

Metabolic techniques for hypothermia are unique in that they induce the body to produce more heat and thus keep itself warmer in the face of a cooling environment. A metabolic technique that has shown the most promise is the intravenous infusion of amino acids to patients undergoing anesthesia. The mechanism by which this increases body heat production is through stimulation of insulin release, which in turn leads to protein synthesis, predominantly in skeletal muscle.[49] Amino acids increase the sensitivity and activity of muscle to the anabolic, muscle-protein synthesis effects of insulin.[50] During muscle-protein synthesis, heat is generated as a by-product and accumulates within the body. The increase in heat production through this mechanism is magnified when an exogenous source of amino acids is administered. Although this technique is not yet recommended for use in a veterinary clinical setting, studies in humans and dogs have demonstrated safety and effectiveness.[51,52]

COMPLICATIONS

Complications associated with using techniques to reduce the severity of IPH are usually associated with the specific technique. Patient skin burns are one of the more severe complications and have been associated with heat lamps or defective or inappropriately operated active technique equipment. Because of the higher risk of burns with heat lamps, they are no longer recommended for use in hypothermic patients. Surgical wound infection can occur with dirty equipment and towels. Infection has been associated with the use of forced warm air blankets that are placed near the surgical field as a result of particles being blown into the surgical field. This can be avoided with proper placement of the blanket and isolation of the surgical field. Reusable blankets should be cleaned between patients and single-use blankets should be disposed of after use on a single patient to prevent nosocomial infections. Circulating warm water pads can leak and harbor infectious agents in the water tanks and should be thoroughly cleaned based on the manufacturer's recommendations.

SUMMARY

IPH is one of the most common complications associated with general anesthesia of dogs and cats. The body's ability to maintain normal temperatures is reduced due to the interactions of anesthetic and analgesic drugs as well as cooling conditions of the perioperative environment. If left untreated, hypothermia can have deleterious effects, including altered pharmacokinetics of anesthetic and analgesic drugs, dysfunction of organ systems, increased patient susceptibility to infection, reduced wound healing, altered coagulation, hypotension, and delayed recovery. Passive and active techniques can be applied to the patient to improve temperature status. Active techniques that apply supplemental heat to the body appear to be most effective.

REFERENCES

1. Torossian A. Thermal management during anaesthesia and thermoregulation standards for the prevention of inadvertent perioperative hypothermia. Best Pract Res Clin Anaesthesiol 2009;22(4):659–68.
2. Satinoff E. Neural organization and evolution of thermal regulation in mammals. Science 1978;201(4350):16–22.
3. Kurz A. Physiology of thermoregulation. Best Pract Res Clin Anaesthesiol 2009; 22(4):627–44.
4. Sessler DI. Temperature regulation and monitoring. In: Miller RD, Cohen NH, Eriksson LI, et al, editors. Miller's anesthesia. 8th edition. St Louis (MO): Saunders Elsevier; 2015. p. 1622–46.
5. Hellyer PW, Roberston SA, Fails AD. Pain and its management. In: Tranquilli WJ, Thurmon JC, Grimm KA, editors. Lumb & Jones' veterinary anesthesia and analgesia. 4th edition. Ames (IA): Blackwell Publishing; 2007. p. 31–57.

6. Hall JE. Body temperature regulation, and fever. In: Hall JE, editor. Guyton and Hall text book of medical physiology. 12th edition. Philadelphia: Saunders Elsevier; 2011. p. 867–77.

7. Hales JR. Skin arteriovenous anastomoses, their control and role in thermoregulation. In: Johansen K, Burggren W, editors. Cardiovascular shunts: phylogenetic, ontogenetic and clinical aspects. Copenhagen (Denmark): Raven Pr; 1986. p. 433–51.

8. Chaplin G, Jablonski NG, Sussman RW, et al. The role of piloerection in primate thermoregulation. Folia Primatol (Basel) 2014;85(1):1–17.

9. Herrington LP. The role of the piliary system in mammals and its relation to the thermal environment. Ann N Y Acad Sci 1951;53(3):600–7.

10. Alfonsi P. Postanaesthetic shivering. Epidemiology, pathophysiology and approaches to prevention and management. Minerva Anestesiol 2003;69:438–41.

11. Ye L, Wu J, Cohen P, et al. Fat cells directly sense temperature to activate thermogenesis. Proc Natl Acad Sci U S A 2013;110(30):12480–5.

12. Blondin DP, Tingelstad HC, Mantha OL, et al. Maintaining thermogenesis in cold exposed humans: Relying on multiple metabolic pathways. Compr Physiol 2014; 4(4):1383–402.

13. Refinetti R, Piccione G. Daily rhythmicity of body temperature in the dog. J Vet Med Sci 2003;65(8):935–7.

14. Osinchuk S, Taylor SM, Shmon CL, et al. Comparison between core temperatures measured telemetrically using the CorTemp® ingestible temperature sensor and rectal temperature in healthy Labrador retrievers. Can Vet J 2014;55(10): 939–45.

15. Taylor NA, Tipton MJ, Kenny GP. Considerations for the measurement of core, skin and mean body temperatures. J Therm Biol 2014;46:72–101.

16. Saritas ZK, Saritas TB, Pamuk K, et al. Comparison of the effects of lidocaine and fentanyl in epidural anesthesia in dogs. Bratisl Lek Listy 2014;115(8):508–13.

17. Vainionpää M, Salla K, Restitutti F, et al. Thermographic imaging of superficial temperature in dogs sedated with medetomidine and butorphanol with and without MK-467 (L-659′066). Vet Anaesth Analg 2013;40(2):142–8.

18. Todd J, Powell LL. Hypothermia. In: Silverstein DC, Hopper K, editors. Small animal critical care medicine. 1st edition. St Louis (MO): Saunders; 2009. p. 720–2.

19. Horosz B, Malec-Milewska M. Inadvertent intraoperative hypothermia. Anaesthesiol Intensive Ther 2013;45(1):38–43.

20. England AL, Wu X, Richards KM, et al. The influences of cold on the recovery of three neuromuscular blocking agents in man. Anaesthesia 1996;51:236–40.

21. Vitez TS, White PF, Eger EI. Effects of hypothermia on halothane MAC and isoflurane MAC in the rat. Anesthesiology 1974;41:80–1.

22. Liu M, Hu X, Liu J. The effect of hypothermia on isoflurane MAC in children. Anesthesiology 2001;94:429–32.

23. Flavahan NA, Lindbalad LE, Verbeuren TJ, et al. Colling and α1- and α2-adrenergic responses in cutaneous veins: role of receptor reserve. Am J Physiol 1985;249(5):H950–5.

24. Weiss SJ, Muniz A, Ernst AA, et al. The physiological response to norepinephrine during hypothermia and rewarming. Resuscitation 1998;39:189–95.

25. Roberts MF, Chilgren JD, Zygmunt AC. Effect of temperature on alpha-adrenoceptor affinity and contractility of rabbit ear blood vessels. Blood Vessels 1989;26:185–96.

26. Kaul SU, Beard DJ, Millar RA. Preganglionic sympathetic activity and baroreceptor responses during hypothermia. Br J Anaesth 1973;45:433–9.

27. Maaravi Y, Weiss AT. The effect of prolonged hypothermia on cardiac function in a young patient with accidental hypothermia. Chest 1990;98(4):1019–20.
28. Goldberg LI. Effects of hypothermia on contractility of the intact dog heart. Am J Physiol 1958;94:92.
29. Moon PF, Ilkiw JE. Surface-induced hypothermia in dogs: 19 cases. J Am Vet Med Assoc 1993;202:437–44.
30. Oncken AK, Kirby R, Rudloff E. Hypothermia in critically ill dogs and cats. Comp Cont Educ Small Anim Pract 2001;23(6):506–21.
31. Stoneham MD, Squires SJ. Prolonged resuscitation in acute deep hypothermia. Anaesthesia 1992;47:784–8.
32. Niwa K, Tasizawa S, Takagi S, et al. Mild hypothermia disturbs regional cerebro-vascular autoregulation in awake rats. Brain Res 1998;789:68–73.
33. Polderman KH. Mechanisms of action, physiological effects, and complications of hypothermia. Crit Care Med 2009;37(7 Suppl):S186–202.
34. de Oliveira JC, de Oliveira CH, de Oliveira HE, et al. Effects of perioperative hypothermia on healing of anastomosis of the colon in rats. Int J Colorectal Dis 2013;28(5):705–12.
35. Du G, Ahao B, Zhang Y, et al. Hypothermia activates adipose tissue to promote malignant lung cancer progression. PLos One 2013;8(8):e72044.
36. Clark-Price SC, Dossin O, Jones KR, et al. Comparison of three different methods to prevent heat loss in healthy dogs undergoing 90 minutes of general anesthesia. Vet Anaesth Analg 2013;40:280–4.
37. Tunsmeyer J, Bojarski I, Nolte I, et al. Intraoperative use of a reflective blanket (Sirius® rescue sheet) for temperature management in dogs less than 10 kg. J Small Anim Pract 2009;50:350–5.
38. Atayde IB, Franco LG, Silva MA, et al. Fluid heating system (SAF): effects on clinical and biochemistry parameters in dogs submitted to inhalatory anesthesia. Acta Cir Bras 2009;24(2):144–9.
39. Cabell LW, Perkowski SZ, Gregor T, et al. The effects of active peripheral skin warming on perioperative hypothermia in dogs. Vet Surg 1997;26:79–85.
40. Evans AT, Sawyer DC, Krahwinkel DJ. Effect of a warm-water blanket on development of hypothermia during small animal surgery. J Am Vet Med Assoc 1973;163: 147–8.
41. Tan C, Govendir CT, Zaki S, et al. Evaluation of four warming procedures to minimize heat loss induced by anaesthesia and surgery in dogs. Aust Vet J 2004;82: 65–8.
42. Nawrocki MA, McLaughlin R, Hendrix PK. The effects of heated and room-temperature abdominal lavage solutions on core body temperature in dogs undergoing celiotomy. J Am Anim Hosp Assoc 2005;41:61–7.
43. Machon RG, Raffe MR, Robinson EP. Warming with a forced air warming blanket minimizes anesthetic-induced hypothermia in cats. Vet Surg 1999;28(4): 301–10.
44. Kinberger O, Held C, Stadelmann K, et al. Resistive polymer versus forced-air warming: comparable heat transfer and core rewarming rates in volunteers. Anesth Analg 2008;107(5):1621–6.
45. Röder G, Sessler DI, Roth G, et al. Intra-operative rewarming with Hot Dog(®) resistive heating and forced-air heating: a trial of lower-body warming. Anesthesia 2011;66(8):667–74.
46. Reed M, Kimberger O, McGovern PD, et al. Forced-air warming design: evaluation of intake filtration, internal microbial buildup, and airborne-contamination emissions. AANA J 2013;81(4):275–80.

47. Wood AM, Moss C, Keenan A, et al. Infection control hazards associated with the use of forced-air warming in operating theatres. J Hosp Infect 2014;88(3):132–40.
48. Malott JC. Hazards of ferrous materials in MRI: a case report. Radiol Technol 1987;58(3):233–5.
49. Yamaoka I, Doi M, Nakayama M, et al. Intravenous administration of amino acids during anesthesia stimulates muscle protein synthesis and heat accumulation in the body. Am J Physiol Endocrinol Metab 2006;290(5):E882–8.
50. Garlick PJ, Grant I. Amino acid infusion increases the sensitivity of muscle protein synthesis in vivo to insulin. Effect of branched-chain amino acids. Biochem J 1988;254(2):579–84.
51. Jin L, Ge S, Wang H, et al. Metabolic effects of intraoperative amino acid infusion in mongrel dogs. Ann Nutr Metab 2012;61:117–25.
52. Clark-Price SC, Dossin O, Ngwenyama TR, et al. The effect of a pre-anesthetic infusion of amino acids on body temperature, venous blood pH, glucose, creatinine, and lactate of healthy dogs during anesthesia. Vet Anaesth Analg 2014; 42(3):299–303.

Postoperative Hemostasis Monitoring and Management

Lisa J. Bazzle, DVM, Benjamin M. Brainard, VMD*

KEYWORDS

- Surgical stress • Hypercoagulability • Venous thromboembolism • Anticoagulant
- Heparin • Aspirin • Bleeding • Bridging

KEY POINTS

- The risk of postoperative venous thromboembolism has been well documented in human medicine, although evidence for its occurrence in veterinary medicine is limited.
- Surgery induces an inflammatory cascade resulting in coagulation activation and disruption, often leading to a transient postoperative hypercoagulable state.
- Diagnosis remains a challenge given the multitude of host- and surgery-related factors that result in a hemostatic seesaw, teetering between thrombosis and hemorrhage.
- Current management relies on careful titration of parenteral and oral anticoagulants that are tailored individually based on risks of thrombosis and bleeding associated with therapy.

INTRODUCTION

Venous thromboembolism (VTE) after surgery is responsible for one-third of the VTE-related human deaths per year in the United States, with pulmonary embolism (PE) as the leading cause of in-hospital mortality.[1] Despite this risk, the ideal thromboprophylactic strategy remains elusive; the timing, type, dose, and duration of anticoagulant therapy is difficult to standardize given the variability of patient condition, surgical procedure, and host response to surgical manipulation. These variables result in inconsistent and sometimes unpredictable responses to anticoagulant therapy.[2] Perioperative monitoring of blood coagulation is important to anticipate not only the risk of thromboembolic events but also to predict the risk of hemorrhage.

Veterinary evidence remains scarce, and even evidence-based recommendations in human medicine lack uniformity, with current practices attempting to reconcile

The authors have nothing to disclose.
Department of Small Animal Medicine and Surgery, College of Veterinary Medicine, University of Georgia, 2200 College Station Road, Athens, GA 30602, USA
* Corresponding author.
E-mail address: brainard@uga.edu

Vet Clin Small Anim 45 (2015) 995–1011
http://dx.doi.org/10.1016/j.cvsm.2015.04.008
0195-5616/15/$ – see front matter © 2015 Elsevier Inc. All rights reserved.

the discrepancies between published studies and clinician experience. Because of this lack of clarity, nearly half of all human patients undergoing major surgery do not receive thromboprophylaxis.[3]

HEMOSTATIC RESPONSE TO SURGICAL STRESS

Inflammation and tissue trauma associated with surgery stimulate a cascade of hormonal, neuroendocrine, metabolic, and hemostatic changes resulting in modulation of immune-derived cytokine release.[4,5] This host-mediated acute phase response may occur locally or systemically and results in at least a 25% change in the concentration of circulating acute phase proteins (APP) and soluble cytokine receptors.[5] The response is characterized by changes in vascular tone and endothelial permeability, serving as an early defense mechanism to control hemorrhage, contain infection, and promote early tissue repair in a controlled manner.

The acute phase response results in elevated levels of fibrinogen and proinflammatory cytokines (eg, tumor necrosis factor alpha [TNF- α], interleukin [IL]-1, and IL-6), which promote leukocyte stimulation and phagocytosis, wound healing and angiogenesis, and stimulation of the hypothalamic-pituitary-adrenal axis.[4] Although the initial acute phase response is generally protective, a prolonged or inappropriately exuberant systemic response can result in pain, immunosuppression, organ dysfunction, thrombohemorrhagic syndromes (ie, disseminated intravascular coagulation [DIC]), or death. This acute phase response can be tracked by the continued increase or delayed decline of serum APP (most have a half-life of 24–48 hours).[4]

Measurable circulating APPs can reflect the severity, invasiveness, and duration of the inflammatory reaction associated with surgery. Prolonged elevations of proinflammatory APPs can induce a hypercoagulable state. Both C-reactive protein (CRP) and serum amyloid A serum concentrations in dogs mirror the resolution of inflammation, even when the total white blood cell count remains elevated, and studies in dogs have found a correlation between CRP levels and surgical trauma.[6,7] Elevated levels of fibrinogen alone may contribute to thromboembolic complications.[8]

SURGICAL STRESS AND POSTOPERATIVE THROMBOPHILIA

Hypercoagulability (or thrombophilia) in the perioperative period is mediated by increased synthesis of APPs, including fibrinogen, CRP, plasminogen activator inhibitor 1 (PAI-1), and increased production of catecholamines and enhanced platelet adhesiveness.[9] Surgical stress stimulates glucocorticoid release, which enhances APP synthesis, which further stimulates the hypothalamic-pituitary-adrenal axis.[10] The cross-talk between inflammation and coagulation is mediated primarily by thrombin, antithrombin (AT), protein C, and the fibrinolytic pathways.[9]

Cytokine induction of a procoagulant state is multifactorial. TNF-α and IL-1β downregulate thrombomodulin, leading to decreased protein C activation and less inhibition of clotting factor activity.[10] IL-1 induces the exposure of tissue factor (TF) on circulating monocytes, which can trigger coagulation at sites of injury or beyond.[11] High levels of IL-6 are associated with increased fibrinogen synthesis, increased thrombin-antithrombin (TAT) complexes, reduced AT activity, and PAI-1 production.[9,11] Increased activity of PAI-1 decreases fibrinolysis, and may result in a prolonged lifespan of clots that have formed.[11,12]

Although all surgical procedures elicit inflammation, the potency of the cytokine response is affected by patient comorbidity, type of surgical procedure, level or type of anesthesia, the surgeon's expertise, and the duration of the procedure.[11,13] Patients undergoing thoracic and abdominal surgery have higher postoperative concentrations of IL-6 and APPs than those undergoing musculoskeletal surgery. Abdominal and thoracic procedures may be associated with greater inflammation, and the peritoneum and splanchnic tissues are rich with macrophages and T cells.[14] During orthopedic surgery, however, bone and joint manipulation causes local TF exposure, in addition to that from soft tissue trauma associated with the procedures. Local activation of coagulation in the venous blood at the site of surgical trauma can result in downstream activation of pulmonary coagulation and fibrinolysis.[15] Certain highly invasive procedures, such as the reaming of the femur associated with total hip replacement have been implicated in the generation of fat emboli, which, although not related to disordered coagulation, can result in ventilation/perfusion mismatching in the lungs and mimic clinical signs of pulmonary thromboembolism in humans and dogs.[16,17]

In horses, fibrinogen and serum amyloid A are more elevated after laparotomy compared with arthroscopic or airway surgery.[18] The same is true in dogs, in which the degree of increase in serum CRP concentration after surgery generally correlates with the degree of tissue trauma.[19] In cats, a 2- to 4-fold increase in various APP has been described in the postoperative period after perineal urethrostomy, castration, or splenectomy.[20,21] The induction of an acute phase response in cats is well described and may be triggered by infectious, endocrine, metabolic, or neoplastic diseases or even by hospitalization alone.[22]

The variability in surgical procedure and invasiveness yields an inconsistent incidence of postoperative VTE in humans (20%–30% after general surgical procedures and 50%–75% after orthopedic operations).[23] In humans undergoing an open surgical procedure, the incidence of fatal PE is between 1% and 5%.[20] The thromboembolic risk with laparoscopic surgery varies between 0.6% and 2.0% and is attributed to venous stasis caused by gas insufflation and pneumoperitoneum.[24,25]

POSTOPERATIVE HYPERCOAGULABILITY IN VETERINARY MEDICINE

In dogs undergoing ovariectomy or ovariohysterectomy, increased fibrinogen and D-dimer concentrations were found in addition to elevations in thromboelastographic (TEG) maximum amplitude (MA), representing clot strength. These patients also displayed a decreased platelet count, von Willebrand factor activity, and factor VIII activity after surgery, with no significant differences between the 2 surgical groups.[26–29] The decreases in platelet count and factor activities are likely caused by consumption from perioperative coagulation needs. Another study in dogs after ovariohysterectomy described significantly prolonged activated partial thromboplastin time (aPTT), elevated fibrinogen and D-dimer concentrations, and lower AT activity 24 hours after surgery, which may also represent consumption and healing.[27] Enhanced fibrinolysis was documented in dogs undergoing ovariohysterectomy and orthopedic surgery through changes in plasma plasminogen and α2-antiplasmin activities.[30]

Decreased AT, protein C, and platelet counts, with an increase in fibrin degradation products, have been found in dogs with bone fractures and thoracic and abdominal trauma and after pancreatic surgery.[31,32] Elevated D-dimer and fibrinogen concentrations as well as decreased protein C and AT activities and increased TEG α angle (representing the rate of clot formation) and MA have been documented perioperatively in dogs with extrahepatic biliary obstruction, although none of these patients were noted to have postoperative thrombosis.[33] Other reports document the presence of PE associated with canine total hip replacement detected via pulmonary perfusion scans although the PE were subclinical in all but one dog and may represent either air, fat, or particles.[34]

Veterinary patients who display hypercoagulability pre- or postoperatively do not necessarily have subsequent thrombosis, and the exact triggering events in most cases are unknown. Until better outcome-focused studies occur in hypercoagulable patients, the determination of which pets are most at risk after surgery remains speculative. Rather than a single test, the best approach for evaluating the postoperative patient is using a comprehensive panel of coagulation assessment (see later discussion) in consideration of the surgical procedure and any patient comorbidities.

COMORBIDITIES THAT CAN EXACERBATE SURGICAL STRESS

Comorbidities can exacerbate hypercoagulable states (**Box 1**). Dogs with sepsis have decreased preoperative concentrations of protein C and AT, predisposing them to hypercoagulability even before the onset of the anticipated surgical inflammation.[10,35] Compounding this trigger is an enhanced rate of bacteremia and systemic inflammation, represented by rapid and sustained increases of IL-1, IL-6, and CRP.[35] These increased proinflammatory cytokines are correlated to elevations in TAT complexes,

---

Box 1
Risk factors for thrombosis

- Central nervous system disease
  - Traumatic brain injury
- Cardiovascular disease
- Respiratory disease
- Gastrointestinal disorders
  - Inflammatory bowel disease
  - Vitamin B deficiency
- Neoplasia
- Hepatobiliary disease
- Nephropathy
- Immune-mediated disease
- Endocrine disease
- Other
  - Obesity
  - Increasing age
  - Anemia
  - Postrenal transplantation
  - Drugs
  - Pregnancy
  - Central venous catheterization
  - Sepsis
  - DIC
  - Hypertension

Data from Refs.[2,33,39,40,43–49,71,110,111]

fibrinogen, and D-dimers. Sepsis or severe sepsis is a common comorbid condition in dogs who display thrombosis in the vena cava or other vessels.[36]

The role of intravenous catheterization on postoperative clot formation must be considered. Many postoperative patients have multiple venous catheters in addition to arterial catheters. The presence of jugular venous catheters has been associated with the formation of cranial vena caval thrombosis in the presence of predisposing factors.[36,37] It is prudent to limit the number of catheters in recovering patients, and the use of multilumen venous catheters can allow intravenous infusion of incompatible medications with a limited number of indwelling catheters. Patients who have had vascular reconstruction or other foreign materials placed into the vascular system (eg, transvenous pacemakers) may have many niduses for the initiation of clot formation that may result in thrombosis or thromboembolism.[37,38] The formation of thrombi on foreign materials in the vascular system likely occurs secondary to endothelial damage and activation of the intrinsic pathway.

Dogs with hyperadrenocorticism have elevated activities or concentrations of coagulation factors II, V, VII, IX, X, XII and fibrinogen, as well as increased circulating TAT complexes and decreased AT, although further studies using other techniques did not necessarily confirm a resting hypercoagulability.[39–41] Thromboembolism as a postoperative event appears to be overrepresented in patients with hyperadrenocorticism or in those treated with corticosteroids, and may be indicative of this exaggerated response.[42,43]

Neoplasia has also been identified as a risk factor for thrombosis in veterinary medicine.[44,45] Thrombosis occurs in 20% of human cancer patients and results in decreased survival and an increased risk of recurrent VTE.[1,46] These effects are thought to be a result of a prothrombotic state secondary to tumor-mediated release of TNF-α and IL-1. Tumors that exhibit vascular invasion may also provide a nidus for clot formation that may result in thromboembolism, and the removal of these tumor thrombi may cause additional endothelial damage to support clot formation. Tumors may also result in a consumptive thrombocytopenia, requiring close monitoring and transfusion support intra- and postoperatively until the platelet count rebounds.

Cardiac disease is an important cause of thromboembolism in cats; abnormal blood flow in the dilated left atria may allow formation of thrombi that can lodge as thromboemboli in either the arterial or venous system.[47] In humans with traumatic brain injury, the risk of deep vein thrombosis development is approximately 20%. This may be caused by the exposure of TF as a result of cerebrovascular disturbances that can trigger a systemic procoagulant state that precedes a hyperfibrinolytic state.[48,49]

DIAGNOSING COAGULATION DISTURBANCES IN THE PERIOPERATIVE SETTING

Coagulation vacillates between thrombosis and fibrinolysis in the postoperative period; the body must maintain clots in areas of surgical wounds, yet cannot break them down too quickly, before tissues have healed. Predicting the risk of thrombosis in a patient population before the introduction of surgical stress may be useful in dictating perioperative hemostasis management. In human medicine, algorithms have been generated to predict the risk of hemorrhage and thrombosis, and some preoperative coagulation testing (activated clotting time and prothrombin time [PT]) weakly correlates with the presence of postoperative coagulopathy.[50] In addition, a persistent consumptive coagulopathy that was present before surgery may result in a hypocoagulable state in the postoperative period.

Traditional plasma assays, such as PT and aPTT, assess the extrinsic and intrinsic clotting cascade respectively; however, these tests are insensitive in identifying the hypercoagulable patient and are more useful to diagnose hypocoagulability.[51] Some studies have associated a shortening of the aPTT with increased thrombin generation, TAT complexes, and D-dimer concentrations.[51–53] In patients who have received significant amounts of intravenous crystalloid or colloid during a surgical procedure, or in those who may have experienced moderate to severe blood loss during surgery, it is indicated to evaluate PT and aPTT in the immediate postoperative period and at least once more in the 12 to 24 hours after surgery. Prolongations of these coagulation times are not generally seen until less than 20% of active coagulation factors are present, and postoperative hypocoagulability should be treated using fresh frozen plasma or fresh whole blood if indicated. Fresh frozen plasma will also provide fibrinogen and other proteins that will support coagulation function. Even if significant hemorrhage did not occur during surgery, patients who have clinical signs of hemorrhagic shock, hemorrhagic drain fluid or effusions, or melena should be evaluated using PT and aPTT with a platelet count. If the patient is suspected to have a consumptive coagulopathy, the measurement of fibrinogen concentration may also help to guide therapy.

Measurement of platelet count provides quantitative information but does not provide information about platelet dysfunction secondary to perioperative, drug-induced, or patient factors. The PFA-100 (Siemens Healthcare USA, Malvern, PA, USA) is a benchtop platelet function analyzer that is easy to use, and may give some information about platelet function in postoperative patients with platelet counts greater than $100 \times 10^3/\mu L$.[54] Monitoring serial platelet counts are important nonetheless. In the postoperative patient, a decreasing platelet count accompanied by a prolonged aPTT may indicate the presence of nonovert DIC. DIC may be present preoperatively but can also develop in the postoperative period. Patients with a significant inflammatory response pre- or postoperatively are at risk for this syndrome, which may result in either hemorrhage or thrombosis. Diagnosis of DIC can be challenging, and beyond the criteria listed above, measurement of fibrinogen or D-dimer concentrations may be helpful. In the authors' experience, patients with sustained inflammation in the postoperative period are the most likely to subsequently have DIC, and efforts should be made to support oxygen delivery and coagulation and to continue to resolve the underlying inflammatory process to correct the condition.

TEG provides information about the viscoelastic properties of clot formation in whole blood and evaluates the entire clotting process, from fibrin formation and maximum clot strength through fibrinolysis. A hypercoagulable state indicated by TEG has been defined as the presence of at least 2 of the following: shortened R time (initial fibrin formation), increased α angle (rate of clot formation), and MA (clot strength).[55] The sensitivity and specificity of TEG for detecting hypercoagulability is variable, and the MA, which indicates the maximum clot strength, is the most reliable parameter to identify hypercoagulability and predict thromboembolic events.[55] Other calculated variables, such as the coagulation index, which combines the R and K times, α angle, and MA into a single number, or the shear elastic modulus strength, which is derived from MA, may offer some insight into the presence or mechanism of hypo- or hypercoagulability. Although many veterinary studies have documented TEG measurements consistent with hypercoagulability, no outcome studies exist at this point that correlate an abnormal TEG to a risk of thrombosis. In patients who display hypocoagulability, TEG has been used to guide transfusion therapy in humans and may be used for this purpose in veterinary medicine as well.[56]

Initial postoperative assessment in most patients with hemorrhage or suspected thrombosis risk should include platelet count, PT, aPTT, fibrinogen concentration, and TEG if available. Ancillary testing such as AT and protein C activity may give additional insight. Subsequent testing should be based on clinical signs or on goal-directed therapy (eg, normalization of coagulation times).

In the otherwise stable patient who starts to bleed after surgery, disorders of fibrinolysis should be considered. A syndrome of delayed postoperative bleeding has been reported in greyhounds and is hypothesized to be secondary to a robust fibrinolytic response.[57] Few tests reliably detect fibrinolysis in veterinary patients. D-dimers are breakdown products of cross-linked fibrin and indicate not only the formation of thrombi but also the body's effort to dissolve the clots. D-dimers may be used as a sentinel of thrombosis, although the sensitivity and specificity of isolated D-dimer measurements in assessing VTE risk in humans and animals is inconsistent. In one veterinary study, D-dimers were significantly higher in patients with known thromboembolism, although concentrations were statistically similar among healthy and ill dogs and dogs after surgery.[58] Another veterinary study found that D-dimers are a poor predictor of pulmonary thromboembolism in dogs.[59] Serial measurement of D-dimers may better elucidate the risk of VTE recurrence; in humans, normal D-dimer concentrations 1 month after discontinuation of anticoagulant therapy were associated with a low risk of recurrence; however, patients who had elevated D-dimer concentrations 3 months after cessation of anticoagulant therapy had a higher risk of recurrence.[60] A recent modification of the TEG to emphasize fibrinolysis has been described but has not been extensively studied in veterinary patients. This modification may represent a more accurate way to interrogate the fibrinolytic pathways in hospitalized patients.[61]

Other advanced methodologies to evaluate for the presence of thrombosis or the activation of coagulation, such as measurement of TAT complexes or flow cytometry to determine the presence of procoagulant microparticles, activated platelets, or platelet-leukocyte aggregates, have been evaluated in research settings in veterinary medicine and offer some tantalizing options to further characterize coagulation in veterinary patients in the near future. The need, however, for advanced equipment and the expense may limit their widespread use.[62–68] TAT complexes have been used for the evaluation of hypercoagulability in human and veterinary medicine, although both serial and isolated measurements have not consistently been associated with increased risk of VTE.[69,70]

PERIOPERATIVE ANTICOAGULANT THERAPY

Thromboprophylaxis, using both mechanical prophylaxis (MP) and pharmacologic prophylaxis, is found to reduce the risk of VTE in humans. MP, including external compressive devices and elastic stockings, results in a 60% to 65% reduction in deep vein thrombosis when compared with no prophylaxis.[71] MP has not been studied in the veterinary population. Pharmacologic prophylaxis in human and veterinary medicine typically includes parenteral anticoagulants with or without oral platelet inhibitors. The timing and type of prophylactic anticoagulation in perioperative patients must balance the risk of thrombosis with that of excessive bleeding.

Parenteral Anticoagulants: Heparins

Unfractionated heparin (UFH) is a heterogeneous, highly sulfated mucopolysaccharide whose binding to AT inactivates thrombin and factors IXa, Xa, XIa, and XIIa. At the time of parenteral injection, heparin binds to several plasma proteins, endothelial cells, macrophages, and von Willebrand factor (most of which are increased or activated by surgery), which can reduce its anticoagulant activity. Heparin's variable binding and metabolism renders its anticoagulant response and half-life variable and nonlinear.[71] Low-dose UFH administered prophylactically to human patients undergoing general, urologic, and orthopedic surgery resulted in an overall mortality reduction of 18%, with a PE and clinical VTE risk reduction of 41% and 70%, respectively. Low-molecular weight heparin (LMWH) reduces risk for PE in a similar population by 66%.[71] UFH has been studied extensively in veterinary medicine and generally requires 3-times-a-day dose administration, although use as a constant rate infusion has also been described.[72,73]

LMWHs are about one-third the molecular weight of UFH and are derived by chemical or enzymatic depolymerization. LMWH has reduced binding to proteins, endothelial cells, and macrophages, and the smaller size renders these molecules unable to inactivate thrombin. LMWHs do inhibit factor Xa, and the anti-Xa to anti-IIa ratio varies between 2:1 and 4:1 (the ratio in UFH is 1:1). Compared with UFH, LMWH has a higher and more predictable subcutaneous (SC) bioavailability (approximately 90%). Because of renal clearance, UFH is recommended over LMWH in patients with severe renal insufficiency.[74] If LMWH is used in patients with renal disease, a 50% dose reduction is recommended to reduce bleeding risks, and anti-Xa monitoring is recommended.[75] The elimination half-life in humans is dose dependent and ranges from 3 to 6 hours after SC injection, with peak anti-Xa levels occurring 3 to 5 hours after dose administration. In veterinary medicine, the pharmacokinetics are less favorable, and LMWHs likely require at least 3-times-a-day dose administration to maintain anticoagulant effect in dogs and cats.[76,77]

The timing of initiation and duration of anticoagulant therapy after surgery remains controversial in people, as the risk of postoperative VTE varies based on the procedure and the patient. The greatest risk of bleeding from anticoagulant therapy is 12 hours before or after surgery, and current human recommendations for LMWH therapy initiate therapy 12 hours after surgery and continue up to 35 days.[78] Despite the elevated risk of VTE extending to 12 weeks after surgery, long-term anticoagulation versus more limited duration thromboprophylaxis (4 weeks) result in the same incidence of symptomatic or fatal VTE.[71]

In patients receiving UFH, monitoring has traditionally been performed using the aPTT, with target prolongations of 1.3 to 1.5 times the baseline. Anti-Xa levels may also be measured. Unactivated TEG is too sensitive to be useful for UFH monitoring, but the use of high-dose (1:3600 final dilution) TF activation may improve the utility of this test.[79,80] LMWHs do not result in significant changes in the PT or aPTT and should be monitored using anti-Xa activity. Target ranges for anti-Xa in humans are 0.5 to 1.0 U/mL for therapeutic uses (ie, treatment of an existing clot) and 0.1 to 0.3 U/mL for prophylactic use. By comparison, the recommended anti-Xa activity for UFH is between 0.35 and 0.7 U/mL for therapeutic uses, with prophylactic uses targeted at 10% of the therapeutic levels.[81,82]

SURGERY-SPECIFIC MODIFICATIONS

Few meta-analyses and randomized controlled studies have been performed to guide prophylaxis of VTE in the surgical patient, and the existing literature is inconsistent and occasionally conflicting regarding superiority of either parenteral anticoagulant over placebo.[83] These findings are further confounded by the variability of dosing regimes and duration of therapy in individual studies. Current human recommendations to target prophylactic levels advocate for once-daily LMWH or low-dose UFH SC 3 times daily starting 12 to 24 hours preoperatively and continuing for at least 7 to 10 days after surgery.[84]

The risk of symptomatic VTE in major orthopedic surgery in humans, specifically total hip and knee arthroplasty, increases from 1.5% immediately postoperatively to

4.3% at 35 days postoperatively. Increases in platelet aggregation and coagulation factor activities can be identified through 7 days after surgery.[85–87] Antiplatelet VTE prophylaxis with low-dose aspirin in human orthopedic patients was found to reduce the incidence of PE by 43% without an increased risk of major bleeding.[50] However, low-dose aspirin is associated with a 50% increase in upper gastrointestinal bleeding, a risk that is dose dependent and reduced with the concurrent administration of proton pump inhibitors.[71,88] The recommendations for low-dose aspirin use in humans apply only to orthopedic surgical patients in cases in which parenteral anticoagulants are contraindicated.[71,89]

Given the low incidence of apparent VTE reported in the veterinary literature, it is difficult to translate these recommendations to the veterinary orthopedic surgery patient, and in the absence of other comorbidities, perioperative anticoagulation is not indicated in this veterinary population. In veterinary patients with significant trauma or inflammation, however, a risk for postoperative thrombosis may be present.[90] It is likely that differences in demographics and early mobility between the human and veterinary groups play a strong role in the difference in VTE occurrence.

RISKS ASSOCIATED WITH ANTICOAGULANT AND THROMBOLYTIC THERAPY

Hemorrhage remains the biggest risk of anticoagulant therapy; however, the effects and quantification of bleeding are not consistently described in human studies, complicating clear interpretation of the risk-to-benefit ratio of perioperative anticoagulant therapy. Even when patients achieve targeted levels of heparin therapy, the risk of hemorrhage remains and is correlated to the heparin dose.

Bleeding risk may be increased with decreased liver or renal function or in patients with acidemia, hypothermia, ionized hypocalcemia, or congenital platelet or clotting factor defects. Concurrent medications (eg, nonsteroidal anti-inflammatory drugs [NSAIDs], antibiotics, thromboprophylactic agents) can also affect bleeding risk. Systematic reviews and meta-analysis in human patients suggest an increased risk of bleeding associated with the invasiveness of the procedure. Overall, there is a 57% increase in nonfatal major bleeding noted in human patients receiving UFH.[71] On initial analysis of studies comparing the difference in VTE risk reduction between LMWH and UFH, the risk of bleeding was 30% lower in the LMWH groups. However, when analysis was restricted to blinded, placebo-controlled trials, no significant difference in clinical PE risk, death, or hemorrhage was noted between LMWH and UFH.[71] The greatest risk of bleeding was in the immediate perioperative period (12 hours before or after surgery), with the lowest risk of bleeding occurring when anticoagulant therapy is instituted more than 24 hours after surgery.[87,91]

PERIOPERATIVE PLANNING

In veterinary species, the use of NSAIDs in the perioperative period has been associated with hemorrhage, although many NSAIDs in current use do not result in irreversible inhibition of platelet function, and the use of more COX-2 selective drugs (eg, coxib-class drugs) may have minimal platelet effects overall.[92]

In humans, the ideal preoperative time to discontinue anticoagulants is complicated by the individual variability of drug pharmacokinetics and the need to balance the risk of hemorrhage with risk of thromboembolism secondary to rapid discontinuation. In many humans receiving long-term warfarin therapy, transition to a shorter-acting anticoagulant drug (ie, UFH, LMWH) is performed for perioperative management because these drugs are easier to manage; this transition is termed *bridging* anticoagulation.[93] Bridging protocols are applied to those patients deemed at high risk for thrombotic events (**Box 2**).[93–97] In this context, and for prophylaxis, LMWH therapy is initiated 2 to 3 days before the procedure, with the last dose given 24 hours before the procedure. Postoperatively, twice daily LMWH is used to avoid high peak concentrations soon after surgery.[95,97]

In human patients receiving long-term antiplatelet therapy, drugs are not always discontinued before surgery. Human studies have shown an increased surgical blood loss of 2.5% to 20% in patients receiving perioperative aspirin, and 30% to 50% with dual antiplatelet therapy (aspirin and clopidogrel), without an increase in surgical mortality.[98] Aspirin remains effective in decreasing thrombotic risk in patients, and an increase in severe bleeding has only been reported for patients undergoing intracranial surgery.[99,100] Patients undergoing peripheral arterial surgery and noncardiac surgery who do not stop antiplatelet medications have a lower risk of myocardial events, whereas abrupt aspirin discontinuation in humans triples the risk of a major cardiovascular event.[101,102] This risk remains to be evaluated in patients undergoing general and abdominal surgery.[103,104] Clopidogrel is associated with a higher incidence of perioperative bleeding compared with aspirin, which may be related to the mechanism of drug action.[71]

No randomized trials exist to determine the optimal time to discontinue aspirin therapy before surgery. Current theories suggest discontinuation of aspirin 7 to 10 days (the lifespan of a circulating platelet) before surgery. However, only 20% of overall platelet function is required for restoration of normal hemostasis, so less overall time may be necessary with the continued production of noninhibited platelets.[71] Platelet aggregometry evaluated in patients after discontinuation of aspirin therapy has found variability in the time required for recovery of adequate platelet function, with longer time required for patients receiving clopidogrel.[105–107] Therefore, continuation of antiplatelet therapy is reserved for patients at high risk of thrombosis, with interruption of drug therapy 2 to 3 half-lives before minor surgery, and 4 to 5 half-lives before major surgery (using the upper limit of the half-life in calculating this time).[108] Otherwise, discontinuation 7 to 10 days preoperatively is recommended.

Box 2
Anticoagulant management recommendations for human surgical patients

High thrombotic risk (>5%)—bridging recommended

- Current treatment for cancer-associated VTE
- Intracranial surgery
- Pneumonectomy
- Trauma, traumatic brain injury
- Orthopedic surgery

Moderate thrombotic risk (3%–5%)—bridging recommended in non–high-risk bleeding procedures + mechanical prophylaxis

- Thoracic, cardiac surgery
- Spinal surgery for malignant disease
- Gynecologic surgery

Low thrombotic risk (<1.5%)—bridging not required

- Same-day/outpatient
- Spinal surgery for nonmalignant disease

Data from Refs.[2,109–111]

Because of the lack of veterinary evidence on discontinuation of antiplatelet medications before surgery, the authors generally apply the human guidelines. For elective surgeries in animals at low risk for thrombosis or thromboembolism, antiplatelet medication may be discontinued 5 to 7 days before the procedures. In animals who have had prior thromboembolism events or who are perceived to be at a higher risk for thromboembolism antiplatelet medications may be continued through surgery or discontinued 48 hours before the start of surgery. Medications may be restarted 24 hours after surgery as long as the patient is not experiencing excessive bleeding or other complications.

SUMMARY

Surgery elicits a potent inflammatory response resulting in a variable thromboembolic risk depending on a multitude of patient- and surgery-related factors. Diagnosis and management of this subsequent hypercoagulable state remains challenging, and further investigation is required to better inform our management decisions to best titrate therapy to maximize reduction of thrombosis with minimal bleeding risk. In the meantime, perioperative anticoagulant and antithrombotic therapy should be considered on an individual basis with simultaneous attempts to reduce intraoperative inflammation, which may include nutritional, hormonal, and supportive fluid therapy in the intraoperative period.

REFERENCES

1. Poredos P, Jezovnik MK. The role of inflammation in venous thromboembolism and the link between arterial and venous thrombosis. Int Angiol 2007;26(4):306–11.
2. Valsami S, Asmis LM. A brief review of 50 years of perioperative thrombosis and hemostasis management. Semin Hematol 2013;50(2):79–87.
3. Bozzato S, Galli L, Ageno W. Thromboprophylaxis in surgical and medical patients. Semin Respir Crit Care Med 2012;33(2):163–75.
4. Cray C, Zaias J, Altman NH. Acute phase response in animals: a review. Comp Med 2009;59(6):517–26.
5. Gabay C, Kushner I. Acute-phase proteins and other systemic responses to inflammation. N Engl J Med 1999;340(6):448–54.
6. Nakamura M, Takahashi M, Ohno K, et al. C-reactive protein concentration in dogs with various diseases. J Vet Med Sci 2008;70(2):127–31.
7. Kjelgaard-Hansen M, Strom H, Mikkelsen LF, et al. Canine serum C-reactive protein as a quantitative marker of the inflammatory stimulus of aseptic elective soft tissue surgery. Vet Clin Pathol 2013;42(3):342–5.
8. Aleman MM, Walton BL, Byrnes JR, et al. Fibrinogen and red blood cells in venous thrombosis. Thromb Res 2014;133(Suppl 1):S38–40.
9. Levi M, van der Poll T, Buller HR. Bidirectional relation between inflammation and coagulation. Circulation 2004;109(22):2698–704.
10. Bentley AM, Mayhew PD, Culp WT, et al. Alterations in the hemostatic profiles of dogs with naturally occurring septic peritonitis. J Vet Emerg Crit Care (San Antonio) 2013;23(1):14–22.
11. Schietroma M, Carlei F, Mownah A, et al. Changes in the blood coagulation, fibrinolysis, and cytokine profile during laparoscopic and open cholecystectomy. Surg Endosc 2004;18(7):1090–6.
12. Tsiminikakis N, Chouillard E, Tsigris C, et al. Fibrinolytic and coagulation pathways after laparoscopic and open surgery: a prospective randomized trial. Surg Endosc 2009;23(12):2762–9.

13. Giannoudis PV, Dinopoulos H, Chalidis B, et al. Surgical stress response. Injury 2006;37(Suppl 5):S3–9.
14. Lin E, Calvano SE, Lowry SF. Inflammatory cytokines and cell response in surgery. Surgery 2000;127(2):117–26.
15. Dahl OE. The role of the pulmonary circulation in the regulation of coagulation and fibrinolysis in relation to major surgery. J Cardiothorac Vasc Anesth 1997; 11(3):322–8.
16. Kosova E, Bergmark B, Piazza G. Fat embolism syndrome. Circulation 2015; 131(3):317–20.
17. Terrell SP, Sundeep Chandra AM, Pablo LS, et al. Fatal intraoperative pulmonary fat embolism during cemented total hip arthroplasty in a dog. J Am Anim Hosp Assoc 2004;40(4):345–8.
18. Jacobsen S, Nielsen JV, Kjelgaard-Hansen M, et al. Acute phase response to surgery of varying intensity in horses: a preliminary study. Vet Surg 2009; 38(6):762–9.
19. Ceron JJ, Eckersall PD, Martynez-Subiela S. Acute phase proteins in dogs and cats: current knowledge and future perspectives. Vet Clin Pathol 2005;34(2): 85–99.
20. Kajikawa T, Furuta A, Onishi T, et al. Changes in concentrations of serum amyloid A protein, alpha 1-acid glycoprotein, haptoglobin, and C-reactive protein in feline sera due to induced inflammation and surgery. Vet Immunol Immunopathol 1999;68(1):91–8.
21. Moldal ER, Kirpensteijn J, Kristensen AT, et al. Evaluation of inflammatory and hemostatic surgical stress responses in male cats after castration under general anesthesia with or without local anesthesia. Am J Vet Res 2012;73(11):1824–31.
22. Paltrinieri S. The feline acute phase reaction. Vet J 2008;177(1):26–35.
23. Milic DJ, Pejcic VD, Zivic SS, et al. Coagulation status and the presence of postoperative deep vein thrombosis in patients undergoing laparoscopic cholecystectomy. Surg Endosc 2007;21(9):1588–92.
24. Dedej T, Lamaj E, Marku N, et al. Alterations in homeostasis after open surgery. A prospective randomized study. G Chir 2013;34(7–8):202–9.
25. Diamantis T, Tsiminikakis N, Skordylaki A, et al. Alterations of hemostasis after laparoscopic and open surgery. Hematology 2007;12(6):561–70.
26. Feige K, Kastner SB, Dempfle CE, et al. Changes in coagulation and markers of fibrinolysis in horses undergoing colic surgery. J Vet Med A Physiol Pathol Clin Med 2003;50(1):30–6.
27. Sobiech P, Targonski R, Stopyra A, et al. Changes in the blood coagulation profile after ovariohysterectomy in female dogs. Pol J Vet Sci 2011;14(2): 289–90.
28. Millis DL, Hauptman JG, Richter M. Preoperative and postoperative hemostatic profiles of dogs undergoing ovariohysterectomy. Cornell Vet 1992;82(4): 465–70.
29. Moldal ER, Kristensen AT, Peeters ME, et al. Hemostatic response to surgical neutering via ovariectomy and ovariohysterectomy in dogs. Am J Vet Res 2012;73(9):1469–76.
30. Lanevschi A, Kramer JW, Greene SA, et al. Fibrinolytic activity in dogs after surgically induced trauma. Am J Vet Res 1996;57(8):1137–40.
31. Mischke R. Acute haemostatic changes in accidentally traumatised dogs. Vet J 2005;169(1):60–4.
32. Alant O, Flautner L, Bock GY, et al. Changes in blood coagulation due to pancreas transplantation in dogs. Acta Chir Acad Sci Hung 1975;16(2):123–30.

33. Mayhew PD, Savigny MR, Otto CM, et al. Evaluation of coagulation in dogs with partial or complete extrahepatic biliary tract obstruction by means of thromboelastography. J Am Vet Med Assoc 2013;242(6):778–85.
34. Liska WD, Poteet BA. Pulmonary embolism associated with canine total hip replacement. Vet Surg 2003;32(2):178–86.
35. Sista F, Schietroma M, Santis GD, et al. Systemic inflammation and immune response after laparotomy vs laparoscopy in patients with acute cholecystitis, complicated by peritonitis. World J Gastrointest Surg 2013;5(4):73–82.
36. Palmer KG, King LG, Van Winkle TJ. Clinical manifestations and associated disease syndromes in dogs with cranial vena cava thrombosis: 17 cases (1989-1996). J Am Vet Med Assoc 1998;213(2):220–4.
37. Singh A, Brisson BA. Chylothorax associated with thrombosis of the cranial vena cava. Can Vet J 2010;51(8):847–52.
38. Cunningham SM, Ames MK, Rush JE, et al. Successful treatment of pacemaker-induced stricture and thrombosis of the cranial vena cava in two dogs by use of anticoagulants and balloon venoplasty. J Am Vet Med Assoc 2009;235(12):1467–73.
39. Jacoby RC, Owings JT, Ortega T, et al. Biochemical basis for the hypercoagulable state seen in Cushing syndrome; discussion 1006-7. Arch Surg 2001; 136(9):1003–6.
40. Klose TC, Creevy KE, Brainard BM. Evaluation of coagulation status in dogs with naturally occurring canine hyperadrenocorticism. J Vet Emerg Crit Care (San Antonio) 2011;21(6):625–32.
41. Pace SL, Creevy KE, Krimer PM, et al. Assessment of coagulation and potential biochemical markers for hypercoagulability in canine hyperadrenocorticism. J Vet Intern Med 2013;27(5):1113–20.
42. Park FM, Blois SL, Abrams-Ogg AC, et al. Hypercoagulability and ACTH-dependent hyperadrenocorticism in dogs. J Vet Intern Med 2013;27(5): 1136–42.
43. Rose L, Dunn ME, Bedard C. Effect of canine hyperadrenocorticism on coagulation parameters. J Vet Intern Med 2013;27(1):207–11.
44. LaRue MJ, Murtaugh RJ. Pulmonary thromboembolism in dogs: 47 cases (1986-1987). J Am Vet Med Assoc 1990;197(10):1368–72.
45. Lake-Bakaar GA, Johnson EG, Griffiths LG. Aortic thrombosis in dogs: 31 cases (2000-2010). J Am Vet Med Assoc 2012;241(7):910–5.
46. Yang Y, Zhou Z, Niu XM, et al. Clinical analysis of postoperative venous thromboembolism risk factors in lung cancer patients. J Surg Oncol 2012;106(6):736–41.
47. Norris CR, Griffey SM, Samii VF. Pulmonary thromboembolism in cats: 29 cases (1987-1997). J Am Vet Med Assoc 1999;215(11):1650–4.
48. Maegele M. Coagulopathy after traumatic brain injury: incidence, pathogenesis, and treatment options. Transfusion 2013;53(Suppl 1):28S–37S.
49. Goh KY, Tsoi WC, Feng CS, et al. Haemostatic changes during surgery for primary brain tumours. J Neurol Neurosurg Psychiatry 1997;63(3):334–8.
50. Collaborative overview of randomised trials of antiplatelet therapy--III: Reduction in venous thrombosis and pulmonary embolism by antiplatelet prophylaxis among surgical and medical patients. Antiplatelet Trialists' Collaboration. BMJ 1994;308(6923):235–46.
51. Jakoi A, Kumar N, Vaccaro A, et al. Perioperative coagulopathy monitoring. Musculoskelet Surg 2014;98(1):1–8.
52. Lipets EN, Ataullakhanov FI. Global assays of hemostasis in the diagnostics of hypercoagulation and evaluation of thrombosis risk. Thromb J 2015;13(1):4 eCollection 2015.

53. Ten Boekel E, Bartels P. Abnormally short activated partial thromboplastin times are related to elevated plasma levels of TAT, F1+2, D-dimer and FVIII: C. Pathophysiol Haemost Thromb 2002;32(3):137–42.

54. Jandrey KE. Assessment of platelet function. J Vet Emerg Crit Care (San Antonio) 2012;22(1):81–98.

55. Park MS, Martini WZ, Dubick MA, et al. Thromboelastography as a better indicator of hypercoagulable state after injury than prothrombin time or activated partial thromboplastin time. J Trauma 2009;67(2):266–75 [discussion: 275–6].

56. Lier H, Vorweg M, Hanke A, et al. Thromboelastometry guided therapy of severe bleeding. Essener Runde algorithm. Hamostaseologie 2013;33(1):51–61.

57. Marin LM, Iazbik MC, Zaldivar-Lopez S, et al. Retrospective evaluation of the effectiveness of epsilon aminocaproic acid for the prevention of postamputation bleeding in retired racing Greyhounds with appendicular bone tumors: 46 cases (2003-2008). J Vet Emerg Crit Care (San Antonio) 2012;22(3):332–40.

58. Nelson OL, Andreasen C. The utility of plasma D-dimer to identify thromboembolic disease in dogs. J Vet Intern Med 2003;17(6):830–4.

59. Epstein SE, Hopper K, Mellema MS, et al. Diagnostic utility of D-dimer concentrations in dogs with pulmonary embolism. J Vet Intern Med 2013;27(6):1646–9.

60. Cosmi B, Legnani C, Tosetto A, et al. Usefulness of repeated D-dimer testing after stopping anticoagulation for a first episode of unprovoked venous thromboembolism: the PROLONG II prospective study. Blood 2010;115(3):481–8.

61. Fletcher DJ, Rozanski EA, Brainard BM, et al. Coagulopathy and hyperfibrinolysis in dogs with spontaneous hemoperitoneum is associated with the severity of shock and depletion of protein C. J Vet Emerg Crit Care, in press.

62. Helmond SE, Catalfamo JL, Brooks MB. Flow cytometric detection and procoagulant activity of circulating canine platelet-derived microparticles. Am J Vet Res 2013;74(2):207–15.

63. Kidd L, Mackman N. Prothrombotic mechanisms and anticoagulant therapy in dogs with immune-mediated hemolytic anemia. J Vet Emerg Crit Care (San Antonio) 2013;23(1):3–13.

64. Maruyama H, Watari T, Miura T, et al. Plasma thrombin-antithrombin complex concentrations in dogs with malignant tumours. Vet Rec 2005;156(26):839–40.

65. Moritz A, Walcheck BK, Weiss DJ. Evaluation of flow cytometric and automated methods for detection of activated platelets in dogs with inflammatory disease. Am J Vet Res 2005;66(2):325–9.

66. Ridyard AE, Shaw DJ, Milne EM. Evaluation of platelet activation in canine immune-mediated haemolytic anaemia. J Small Anim Pract 2010;51(6):296–304.

67. Weiss DJ, Brazzell JL. Detection of activated platelets in dogs with primary immune-mediated hemolytic anemia. J Vet Intern Med 2006;20(3):682–6.

68. Wills TB, Wardrop KJ, Meyers KM. Detection of activated platelets in canine blood by use of flow cytometry. Am J Vet Res 2006;67(1):56–63.

69. Ginsberg JS, Brill-Edwards P, Panju A, et al. Pre-operative plasma levels of thrombin-antithrombin III complexes correlate with the development of venous thrombosis after major hip or knee surgery. Thromb Haemost 1995;74(2):602–5.

70. Pazzagli M, Mazzantini D, Cella G, et al. Value of thrombin-antithrombin III complexes in major orthopedic surgery: relation to the onset of venous thromboembolism. Clin Appl Thromb Hemost 1999;5(4):228–31.

71. Gould MK, Garcia DA, Wren SM, et al. Prevention of VTE in nonorthopedic surgical patients: antithrombotic therapy and prevention of thrombosis, 9th ed:

American College of Chest Physicians evidence-based clinical practice guidelines. Chest 2012;141(2 Suppl):e227S–77S.

72. Babski DM, Brainard BM, Ralph AG, et al. Sonoclot(R) evaluation of single- and multiple-dose subcutaneous unfractionated heparin therapy in healthy adult dogs. J Vet Intern Med 2012;26(3):631–8.

73. Scott KC, Hansen BD, DeFrancesco TC. Coagulation effects of low molecular weight heparin compared with heparin in dogs considered to be at risk for clinically significant venous thrombosis. J Vet Emerg Crit Care (San Antonio) 2009; 19(1):74–80.

74. Geerts WH, Bergqvist D, Pineo GF, et al. Prevention of venous thromboembolism: American College of Chest Physicians evidence-based clinical practice guidelines (8th edition). Chest 2008;133(6 Suppl):381S–453S.

75. Lynch AM, deLaforcade AM, Sharp CR. Clinical experience of anti-Xa monitoring in critically ill dogs receiving dalteparin. J Vet Emerg Crit Care (San Antonio) 2014;24(4):421–8.

76. Brainard BM, Koenig A, Babski DM, et al. Viscoelastic pharmacodynamics after dalteparin administration to healthy dogs. Am J Vet Res 2012;73(10):1577–82.

77. Alwood AJ, Downend AB, Brooks MB, et al. Anticoagulant effects of low-molecular-weight heparins in healthy cats. J Vet Intern Med 2007;21(3):378–87.

78. Falck-Ytter Y, Francis CW, Johanson NA, et al. Prevention of VTE in orthopedic surgery patients: antithrombotic therapy and prevention of thrombosis, 9th ed: American College of Chest Physicians evidence-based clinical practice guidelines. Chest 2012;141(2 Suppl):e278S–325S.

79. Pittman JR, Koenig A, Brainard BM. The effect of unfractionated heparin on thrombelastographic analysis in healthy dogs. J Vet Emerg Crit Care (San Antonio) 2010;20(2):216–23.

80. Brainard B, Koenig A, Pittman J, et al. Evaluation of high-dose tissue-factor activated thrombelastography for assessment of unfractionated and low molecular weight heparin therapy in dogs. J Vet Emerg Crit Care 2011;21:S10–1.

81. Hirsh J, Bauer KA, Donati MB, et al. Parenteral anticoagulants: American College of Chest physicians evidence-based clinical practice guidelines (8th edition). Chest 2008;133(6 Suppl):141S–59S.

82. Brainard BM, Brown AJ. Defects in coagulation encountered in small animal critical care. Vet Clin North Am Small Anim Pract 2011;41(4):783–803.

83. Akl EA, Kahale L, Sperati F, et al. Low molecular weight heparin versus unfractionated heparin for perioperative thromboprophylaxis in patients with cancer. Cochrane Database Syst Rev 2014;(6):CD009447.

84. Farge D, Debourdeau P, Beckers M, et al. International clinical practice guidelines for the treatment and prophylaxis of venous thromboembolism in patients with cancer. J Thromb Haemost 2013;11(1):56–70.

85. Lopez Y, Paramo JA, Valenti JR, et al. Hemostatic markers in surgery: a different fibrinolytic activity may be of pathophysiological significance in orthopedic versus abdominal surgery. Int J Clin Lab Res 1997;27(4):233–7.

86. Oberweis BS, Cuff G, Rosenberg A, et al. Platelet aggregation and coagulation factors in orthopedic surgery. J Thromb Thrombolysis 2014;38(4):430–8.

87. Solayar GN, Shannon FJ. Thromboprophylaxis and orthopaedic surgery: options and current guidelines. Malays J Med Sci 2014;21(3):71–7.

88. Valkhoff VE, Sturkenboom MC, Hill C, et al. Low-dose acetylsalicylic acid use and the risk of upper gastrointestinal bleeding: a meta-analysis of randomized clinical trials and observational studies. Can J Gastroenterol 2013;27(3):159–67.

89. Prevention of pulmonary embolism and deep vein thrombosis with low dose aspirin: Pulmonary Embolism Prevention (PEP) trial. Lancet 2000;355(9212):1295–302.

90. DePaula KM, deLaorcade AM, King RG, et al. Arterial thrombosis after vehicular trauma and humeral fracture in a dog. J Am Vet Med Assoc 2013;243(3):394–8.

91. Mismetti P, Laporte S, Darmon JY, et al. Meta-analysis of low molecular weight heparin in the prevention of venous thromboembolism in general surgery. Br J Surg 2001;88(7):913–30.

92. Brainard BM, Meredith CP, Callan MB, et al. Changes in platelet function, hemostasis, and prostaglandin expression after treatment with nonsteroidal anti-inflammatory drugs with various cyclooxygenase selectivities in dogs. Am J Vet Res 2007;68(3):251–7.

93. van Veen JJ, Makris M. Management of peri-operative anti-thrombotic therapy. Anaesthesia 2015;70(Suppl 1):58–67 e21–3.

94. Pither C, Middleton S, Gao R, et al. Prothrombotic disorders in a cohort of 25 patients undergoing transplantation: investigation and management implications. Transplant Proc 2014;46(6):2133–5.

95. Dunn AS, Spyropoulos AC, Turpie AG. Bridging therapy in patients on long-term oral anticoagulants who require surgery: the Prospective Peri-operative Enoxaparin Cohort Trial (PROSPECT). J Thromb Haemost 2007;5(11):2211–8.

96. Spyropoulos AC, Turpie AG, Dunn AS, et al. Clinical outcomes with unfractionated heparin or low-molecular-weight heparin as bridging therapy in patients on long-term oral anticoagulants: the REGIMEN registry. J Thromb Haemost 2006;4(6):1246–52.

97. Tafur AJ, McBane R 2nd, Wysokinski WE, et al. Predictors of major bleeding in peri-procedural anticoagulation management. J Thromb Haemost 2012;10(2):261–7.

98. Payne DA, Hayes PD, Jones CI, et al. Combined therapy with clopidogrel and aspirin significantly increases the bleeding time through a synergistic antiplatelet action. J Vasc Surg 2002;35(6):1204–9.

99. Sun JC, Whitlock R, Cheng J, et al. The effect of pre-operative aspirin on bleeding, transfusion, myocardial infarction, and mortality in coronary artery bypass surgery: a systematic review of randomized and observational studies. Eur Heart J 2008;29(8):1057–71.

100. Burger W, Chemnitius JM, Kneissl GD, et al. Low-dose aspirin for secondary cardiovascular prevention - cardiovascular risks after its perioperative withdrawal versus bleeding risks with its continuation - review and meta-analysis. J Intern Med 2005;257(5):399–414.

101. Oscarsson A, Gupta A, Fredrikson M, et al. To continue or discontinue aspirin in the perioperative period: a randomized, controlled clinical trial. Br J Anaesth 2010;104(3):305–12.

102. Vaclavik J, Taborsky M. Antiplatelet therapy in the perioperative period. Eur J Intern Med 2011;22(1):26–31.

103. Antolovic D, Reissfelder C, Rakow A, et al. A randomised controlled trial to evaluate and optimize the use of antiplatelet agents in the perioperative management in patients undergoing general and abdominal surgery–the APAP trial (ISRCTN45810007). BMC Surg 2011;11:7.

104. Lordkipanidze M, Diodati JG, Pharand C. Possibility of a rebound phenomenon following antiplatelet therapy withdrawal: a look at the clinical and pharmacological evidence. Pharmacol Ther 2009;123(2):178–86.

105. Le Manach Y, Kahn D, Bachelot-Loza C, et al. Impact of aspirin and clopidogrel interruption on platelet function in patients undergoing major vascular surgery. PLoS One 2014;9(8):e104491.
106. Li C, Hirsh J, Xie C, et al. Reversal of the anti-platelet effects of aspirin and clopidogrel. J Thromb Haemost 2012;10(4):521–8.
107. Zisman E, Erport A, Kohanovsky E, et al. Platelet function recovery after cessation of aspirin: preliminary study of volunteers and surgical patients. Eur J Anaesthesiol 2010;27(7):617–23.
108. Spyropoulos AC, Douketis JD. How I treat anticoagulated patients undergoing an elective procedure or surgery. Blood 2012;120(15):2954–62.
109. Douketis JD, Spyropoulos AC, Spencer F, et al. Perioperative management of antithrombotic therapy: Antithrombotic Therapy and Prevention of Thrombosis, 9th ed: American College of Chest Physicians Evidence-Based Clinical Practice Guidelines. Chest 2012;141(2 Suppl):e326S–50S.
110. Antiel RM, Hashim Y, Moir CR, et al. Intra-abdominal venous thrombosis after colectomy in pediatric patients with chronic ulcerative colitis: incidence, treatment, and outcomes. J Pediatr Surg 2014;49(4):614–7.
111. Lim W, Meade M, Lauzier F, et al. Failure of anticoagulant thromboprophylaxis: risk factors in medical-surgical critically ill patients. Crit Care Med 2015;43(2):401–10.

Analgesia in the Perioperative Period

Stephanie H. Berry, DVM, MS

KEYWORDS

- Pain • Analgesia • Perioperative • Dog • Cat

KEY POINTS

- Untreated or undermanaged perioperative pain has adverse welfare and systemic effects.
- A patient's pain and comfort should be assessed at regular intervals during the perioperative period.
- Validated pain assessment tools are available for use in dogs and cats.
- Multimodal analgesic plans should be created for individual patients and modified according to pain assessments.
- The gold standard of pain assessment is response to analgesic therapy. If in doubt, administer analgesics.

INTRODUCTION

Effective management of pain in the perioperative period remains challenging despite the recognition of its importance to patient welfare and healing. Difficulty in accurately diagnosing and assessing pain, and unfamiliarity with available analgesic drugs and techniques likely contribute to the undermanagement of perioperative pain in veterinary patients.

WHY SHOULD I TREAT PERIOPERATIVE PAIN?

An understanding of the physiology and pathophysiology of pain leaves little doubt that untreated pain results in many untoward physiologic responses involving all body systems. Some of the potential consequences of untreated perioperative pain are described next based on the body system affected[1]:

- Cardiovascular: tachycardia; increased systemic vascular resistance; increased oxygen consumption by the myocardium; altered blood flow, which may impair wound healing; hypercoagulability

The author has nothing to disclose.
Department of Companion Animals, Atlantic Veterinary College, 550 University Avenue, Charlottetown, Prince Edward Island C1A 4P3, Canada
E-mail address: sberry@upei.ca

- Respiratory: splinting of chest wall muscles and diaphragm resulting in decreased tidal volume, hypoventilation, hypoxemia
- Gastrointestinal: decreased motility and delays in gastric emptying, decreased perfusion leading to bacterial translocation and possibly sepsis
- Neuroendocrine: increased catabolic hormones leading to catabolic state and impaired wound healing and muscle wasting
- Nervous: stress, anxiety, fear, and aggression

HOW DO I DETERMINE IF MY PATIENT IS IN PAIN?

Veterinary patients depend on the veterinarian to anticipate, recognize, and assess the presence of pain. Assessment of pain in dogs and cats should be performed as a part of the physical examination and at regular intervals during the perioperative period.

Practitioners and caregivers should be familiar with behaviors that may be associated with pain in the dog and cat. Dogs in pain may exhibit the following behaviors[2]:

- Change in posture: holding tail between legs, arching of the back, or drooping of the head
- Changes in mobility: reluctance to move, lameness
- Changes in temperament: attacking, biting
- Barking, whimpering
- Inappetence

Cats may show more subtle signs of pain including the following:

- Reduced interaction with people: escaping, hiding[3]
- Reluctance to move[3]
- Change in facial expression: squinting of eyes, furrowed brow[4]
- Reduction in grooming and appetite[3]

Assessment tools are also available to assist the practitioner. These include one-dimensional scales (eg, visual analogue, simple descriptive, and numerical rating scales) and composite scales, some of which have been validated in small animal patients (**Table 1**). The practitioner should become familiar with these behaviors and tools and use them consistently when evaluating patients. Consistent and rigorous

Table 1
Assessment tools available for use in the dog and cat

Species	Tool	Source	Validated
Dog	University of Glasgow Short Form Composite Pain Score	http://www.newmetrica.com/cmps/	Yes
	4A-VET	http://www.medvet.umontreal.ca/4avet/	—
	Colorado State University Canine Acute Pain Scale	http://www.csuanimalcancercenter.org/assets/files/csu_acute_pain_scale_canine.pdf	—
Cat	UNESP-Botucatu multidimensional composite pain scale	http://www.animalpain.com.br/en-us/avaliacao-da-dor-em-gatos.php	Yes
	Colorado State University Feline Acute Pain Scale	http://www.csuanimalcancercenter.org/assets/files/csu_acute_pain_scale_feline.pdf	—

use of pain assessments reduces subjectivity, decreases bias, and improves the effectiveness of the analgesic plan.

Whichever assessment tool is incorporated into practice, some basic principles should be remembered:

- Assessment should always include a thorough history and physical examination.
- Assessments should be performed on an individual basis, because there are no universal analgesic protocols that work for all types of pain or surgical procedure.
- Animals should be assessed from a distance at first. Then the observer should approach and interact with the animal, palpating the painful area if possible.
- The frequency of the assessments depends on the anticipated severity and duration of pain, and the expected duration of the analgesic technique.
- The gold standard in pain assessment is the response to treatment. If in doubt, analgesics should be administered and the patient reassessed.

HOW DO I CREATE AN ANALGESIC PLAN?

Analgesic plans should strive to be preventative, multimodal, and flexible. Several studies in human and veterinary patients demonstrate that administration of analgesics, particularly nonsteroidal anti-inflammatory drugs (NSAIDs), local anesthetics, and epidural injections before surgery may improve pain scores and reduce the amount of analgesia needed postoperatively.[5–8]

Analgesic plans comprised of different classes of analgesic drugs and techniques are known as multimodal or balanced analgesic plans. The goal of a multimodal plan should be to incorporate drugs or therapies that act on different areas of the pain pathway and work synergistically. A balanced plan ideally enables lower doses of each analgesic drug and thus limits adverse effects. The list of available analgesic drugs and techniques can be overwhelming when considered individually; however, an effective multimodal plan can usually be created by the following steps (**Fig. 1**):

1. Choose an opioid
2. Choose a NSAID (unless contraindicated)
3. Incorporate a local anesthetic
4. Decide if administration of an α_2-agonist would benefit the patient
5. Choose analgesic adjuncts (eg, ketamine, gabapentin) if needed
6. Use nonpharmacologic techniques to minimize pain

WHICH OPIOID DO I CHOOSE?

In almost all cases, opioids form the base of a balanced analgesic plan. Opioids used in the management of perioperative pain are found in **Table 2**. Opioids are classified by their affinity for and action at specific opioid receptors (mu, kappa, delta, nociceptin). These receptors are found in varying densities throughout the brain, spinal cord, and peripheral tissues. Activation of the opioid receptor results in a decrease in the release of excitatory neurotransmitters and a hyperpolarization of neurons with the overall effect being an inhibition of painful stimuli transmission.

Choice of opioid is based on the knowledge of the patient, procedure, and expected degree and duration of pain. Commonly, mu agonist opioids (eg, morphine, fentanyl) are chosen for treatment of moderate to severe pain, whereas partial mu agonists (eg, buprenorphine) are used when moderate pain is expected. The mixed kappa agonist/mu antagonist, butorphanol, is usually only recommended for mildly painful patients or procedures. Side effects of opioid administration include bradycardia, respiratory

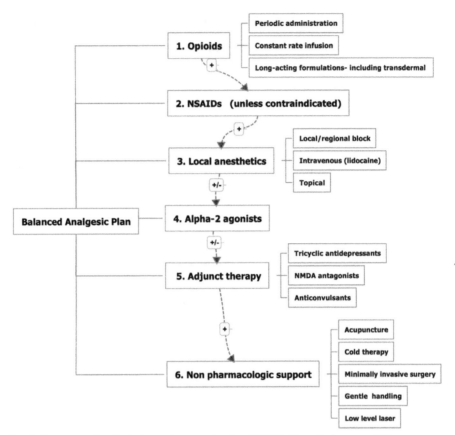

Fig. 1. Components of a balanced analgesic plan. NMDA, *N*-methyl-D-aspartate.

depression, tachypnea, emesis, nausea, sedation, dysphoria, and altered thermoregulation. These side effects are more likely to occur with excessive doses, but should be considered when constructing an analgesic plan.

Once an opioid is selected, the clinician should determine the method of administration. Options include intermittent parenteral administration; constant rate infusion; or, with some opioids, long-acting formulations are available.

A long-acting topically applied form of fentanyl (Recuvyra) has recently been approved for use in dogs. It is applied to the skin 2 to 4 hours before surgery with a needleless application system and dries rapidly. The fentanyl is absorbed quickly and sequestered in the stratum corneum where it is slowly absorbed into the blood.[9] A single application applied to the interscapular skin of beagles resulted in plasma concentrations consistent with analgesia 4 hours after administration and lasting for 96 hours.[10] When compared with intermittent injection of other opioids (buprenorphine and oxymorphone), this formulation was found to be effective and safe.[11,12] It should also be noted that the opioid antagonist naloxone was able to reverse the effects of overdose when administered at hourly intervals.[13] Because this product is approved for dogs and reduces the chance for accidental human exposure, it is recommended that it be used in place of the commercially available human transdermal patches.

Table 2
Opioids used in the dog and cat

Type	Drug	Dosage for Dogs	Dosage for Cats	Notes
Full mu agonists	Morphine (Morphine)	0.05–0.1 mg/kg IV q 1–2 h 0.05–0.1 mg/kg/h IV CRI 0.5–1.0 mg/kg IM q 3–5 h 0.1 mg/kg epidural q 12–24 h	0.05–0.1 mg/kg IV q 1–2 h 0.05–0.1 mg/kg/h IV CRI 0.1–0.2 mg/kg IM q 3–4 h 0.1 mg/kg epidural q 12–24 h	Can produce dysphoria in cats with higher doses Histamine release when given IV
	Hydromorphone (Dilaudid)	0.05–0.1 mg/kg IV q 1–2 h 0.05–0.1 mg/kg/h IV CRI 0.1–0.2 mg/kg IM q 3–4 h	0.05–0.1 mg/kg IV q 1–2 h 0.01–0.05 mg/kg/h IV CRI 0.05–0.1 mg/kg IM q 3–4 h	Associated with occasional hyperthermia in cats No histamine release with IV administration Less emesis than morphine
	Oxymorphone (Numorphan)	0.05–0.1 mg/kg IV, IM q 4 h	0.05–0.1 mg/kg IV, IM q 4 h	—
	Fentanyl (Sublimaze)	0.01–0.04 mg/kg IM q 30 min 0.002–0.005 mg/kg IV 0.002–0.02 mg/kg/h IV CRI	0.005–0.02 mg/kg IM q 30 min 0.002–0.005 mg/kg IV 0.002–0.02 mg/kg/h IV CRI	—
	Fentanyl (Recuvyra)	2.7 mg/kg topical Duration is at least 96 h	Not approved	Approved for use in the dog Must be trained in application before using
	Remifentanil (Ultiva)	0.004–0.01 mg/kg IV 0.004–0.012 mg/kg/h IV CRI	0.004–0.006 mg/kg IV 0.004–0.006 mg/kg/h IV CRI	Constant rate infusion does not require a loading dose
	Methadone (Dolophine)	0.1–0.5 mg/kg IV, IM q 2–4 h	0.1–0.25 mg/kg IV, IM q 2–4 h 0.1–0.3 mg/kg OTM q 8–12 h	—
Partial mu agonist	Buprenorphine (Buprenex)	0.005–0.02 mg/kg IV, IM q 4–8 h	0.005–0.02 mg/kg IV, IM q 4–8 h 0.02–0.04 mg/kg OTM q 4–8 h	Onset of action may be 30 min or more
	Buprenorphine (Simbadol)	Not approved	0.24 mg/kg SC q 24 h	Administer 1 h before surgery Continue daily dosing for 3 d
Kappa agonist/mu antagonist	Butorphanol (Torbugesic)	0.2–0.4 mg/kg IV, IM q 1 h	0.2–0.4 mg/kg IV, IM q 1 h	—
Mixed mechanism mu agonists	Tramadol (Ultram)	1–4 mg/kg IV q 6–8 h	1–4 mg/kg IV q 6–8 h	—
	Tapentadol (Nucynta)	2–6 mg/kg IV	—	—

Abbreviations: CRI, constant rate infusion; IM, intramuscularly; IV, intravenously; OTM, oral transmucosal; SC, subcutaneously.

The partial mu agonist buprenorphine is commonly used to provide analgesia in cats. A recent review of the literature involving buprenorphine administration in cats determined that the route of administration affects the onset, duration, and amount of analgesia, with subcutaneous administration resulting in inadequate analgesia.[14] Buccal administration of buprenorphine produced inconsistent levels of analgesia, whereas the intramuscular and intravenous routes seem to be superior.[14] A sustained-release formulation of buprenorphine (Simbadol) has recently been approved for use in cats. It is recommended that the product be given subcutaneously approximately 1 hour before surgery and then once every 24 hours for up to 3 days.[15] Studies of cats undergoing soft tissue or orthopedic surgery showed that this formulation of buprenorphine was more effective than placebo at controlling pain.[15] Side effects of administration included a decrease in respiratory rate and mean arterial blood pressure during general anesthesia.[15] Although further studies using this formulation of buprenorphine in clinical settings would be beneficial, this remains the only sustained-release buprenorphine that has received approval from the Food and Drug Administration.

Tramadol and Tapentadol

Tramadol produces analgesia by activation of mu opioid receptors, facilitation of serotonin release, and inhibition of norepinephrine reuptake.[16] The injectable form of the drug has been shown to provide adequate analgesia in dogs experiencing mild to moderate levels of pain.[17,18] In cats undergoing ovariohysterectomy, injectable tramadol combined with an NSAID provided adequate analgesia[19] and oral administration increased thermal thresholds.[20] Side effects of tramadol administration include bradycardia, nausea, and constipation or diarrhea.

Tapentadol is a novel analgesic that produces this effect by activation of the mu opioid receptors and inhibition of the reuptake of norepinephrine.[21] One study using tapentadol in an acute pain model in the dog has been published.[22] Tapentadol was administered to beagles and found to produce potent antinociception.[22] Interestingly, when using the same model, tramadol did not induce any antinociception in contrast to many reported studies.[22] To the author's knowledge, there are no publications describing the use of tapentadol in cats.

CHOOSING A NONSTEROIDAL ANTI-INFLAMMATORY DRUG

Patients in the perioperative period primarily suffer from acute inflammatory pain resulting from activation of the immune system caused by tissue injury. The pain begins suddenly and lasts until healing has occurred. Because of the inflammatory component of perioperative pain, NSAIDs play an important role in the management of mild to moderate pain in these patients and should be included in a balanced analgesic plan if possible.

NSAIDs act by inhibiting cyclooxygenase enzymes, which decreases the release of prostanoids and prostaglandin.[23] These drugs produce analgesia, anti-inflammatory, and antipyretic effects at the site of tissue injury and at the level of the central nervous system.[24] Gastrointestinal side effects ranging from gastritis and vomiting to intestinal perforation, hemorrhage, and death have been reported.[25] Nephrotoxicity and hepatotoxicity have also been documented.[26,27] NSAIDs should be used with caution, or avoided in patients with

- Hypovolemia, dehydration, hypotension, shock
- Renal or hepatic insufficiency
- Congestive heart failure, cardiac dysfunction

- Gastric ulcers
- Coagulopathy
- Concurrent administration of nephrotoxic drugs, other NSAIDs, or corticosteroids

Careful and regular monitoring for gastrointestinal, renal, and/or hepatic toxicity should be performed when using this class of drugs. NSAIDs commonly used in perioperative analgesic plans are listed in **Table 3**.

HOW CAN I INCORPORATE A LOCAL ANESTHETIC?

Local anesthetics are inexpensive, easy to use, and rarely associated with significant adverse events. They are incorporated into a balanced analgesic plan in several ways and it is recommended that they be included in the plan of every surgical patient.[28] Local anesthetics prevent the conduction and propagation of nerve impulses by binding to voltage-gated sodium channels, producing complete analgesia.[29] Adverse events associated with local anesthetic administration are usually the result of inadvertent intravenous administration (bupivacaine) or overdose. Signs of local anesthetic toxicity include ataxia; nystagmus; and tremors, which can progress to convulsions, unconsciousness, and respiratory arrest.[30] Cardiovascular manifestations of local

Table 3			
NSAIDs used for the treatment of acute pain in the dog and cat			
Drug	**Dosage in the Dog**	**Dosage in the Cat**	**Notes**
Carprofen (Rimadyl)	4.4 mg/kg IV, SC once 2.2 mg/kg PO q 12 h 4.4 mg/kg PO q 24 h	1–4 mg/kg IV, SC once	Oral administration in the dog for up to 4 d
Deracoxib (Deramaxx)	3–4 mg/kg PO q 24 h	—	Once daily for 7 d
Cimicoxib (Cimalgex)	2 mg/kg PO q 24 h	—	Once daily for 4–8 d
Ketoprofen (Ketofen)	1–2 mg/kg IV, IM, SC once 1 mg/kg PO q 24 h for up to 3 d	0.5–2 mg/kg IV, IM, SC once 0.5–1 mg/kg PO q 24 h for up to 3 d	—
Meloxicam (Metacam)	0.2 mg/kg IV, SC once 0.1 mg/kg PO q 24 h	0.3 mg/kg SC once	—
Firocoxib (Previcox)	5 mg/kg PO q 24 h for 3 d	—	—
Robenacoxib (Onsior)	2 mg/kg SC once 1 mg/kg PO q 24 h	2 mg/kg SC q 24 h 1 mg/kg PO q 24 h	—
Ketorolac (Toradol)	0.5 mg/kg IV, IM, SC q 12 h	0.2 mg/kg IM q 12 h	Use for one to two treatments
Acetaminophen (Tylenol, generic)	10–15 mg/kg PO q 8–12 h	Do not use	—
Aspirin (generic)	10–25 mg/kg PO q 8–12 h	10–25 mg/kg PO q 48 h	—
Tolfenamic acid (Tolfedine, Vetoquinol)	4 mg/kg IM, SC, PO q 24 h Give for 4 d, then off for 3 d	4 mg/kg IM, SC, PO q 24 h for 3 d	—

Abbreviations: IM, intramuscularly; IV, intravenously.

anesthetic toxicity include bradycardia and sinus arrest.[31] The versatility of local anesthetics allows them to be used in several ways:

- Topical: local anesthetics can be applied to skin or mucosa to desensitize areas (eg, lidocaine spray, lidocaine patch)
- Infiltrative: local anesthetics can be injected near specific nerves or placed in wounds (eg, peripheral nerve blocks, soaker catheters)
- Systemic: lidocaine may be given intravenously to dogs to decrease inhaled anesthetic requirements and provide anti-inflammatory effects
- Neuraxial: intrathecal or epidural application of local anesthetics

Table 4 lists commonly used local anesthetics, and **Table 5** describes some of the various ways these drugs can be used to provide analgesia.

WOULD AN α_2-AGONIST BE HELPFUL?

α_2-Agonist receptors are located in close proximity to opioid receptors throughout the body. Therefore, when opioids and α_2-agonists are used concurrently as part of a balanced analgesic plan, there is a synergistic effect with sedation and analgesia. It should be remembered that drugs of this class have significant effects on the cardiovascular and respiratory systems. Cardiovascular effects include bradycardia, hypertension, hypotension, reduction in cardiac output, and stroke volume.[32] A reduction in respiratory rate and tidal volume are also seen, which may result in respiratory acidosis and hypoxemia in some animals.[33] These effects can be seen even when very small doses of α_2-agonists are administered, therefore their use should be limited to those animals that can tolerate derangements of the cardiovascular and respiratory systems (eg, those without significant systemic disease).

Table 4
Local anesthetics used for the treatment of acute pain in the dog and cat

Drug	Onset	Duration	Dosage in the Dog	Dosage in the Cat
Lidocaine (Lidocaine)	5–10 min	1–3 h	2 mg/kg IV 0.025–0.05 mg/kg/min IV CRI 4.4 mg/kg epidural Maximum recommended dose: 8 mg/kg	Constant rate infusion not recommended in the cat[52] 4.4 mg/kg epidural Maximum recommended dose: 6 mg/kg
Mepivacaine (Carbocaine V)	3–10 min	2–4 h	Maximum recommended dose: 4.5 mg/kg	Maximum recommended dose: 3 mg/kg
Bupivacaine (Marcaine)	10–20 min	3–6 h	1–1.5 mg/kg epidural Maximum recommended dose: 2 mg/kg	1 mg/kg epidural Maximum recommended dose: 1 mg/kg
Etidocaine (Duranest)	3–5 min	5–10 h	Maximum recommended dose: 8 mg/kg	Maximum recommended dose: 4 mg/kg
Ropivicaine (Naropin)	15–20 min	1.5–6 h	0.5 mg/kg epidural Maximum recommended dose: 3 mg/kg	0.5 mg/kg epidural Maximum recommended dose: 1.5 mg/kg

Abbreviations: CRI, constant rate infusion; IV, intravenously.

Table 5 Common methods to incorporate local anesthetics into analgesic protocols	
Area of Body Effected	**Local Anesthetic Technique**
Head	Selective nerve blocks (eg, inferior alveolar, maxillary)
Forelimb	Paravertebral forelimb block Brachial plexus block Proximal RUMM block Distal RUM Intravenous regional anesthesia
Thorax	Intercostal nerve blocks Intrapleural injection Epidural injection
Abdomen	Transverse abdominis plane block[53] Epidural injection Intrapleural injection
Hind limb	Selective nerve blocks (eg, femoral) Epidural injection
Testicle/ovary	Intratesticular injection Infiltration of ovarian ligament
Wounds/incisions	Infiltration Diffusion catheter[54] Transdermal patch
Joints	Intra-articular injection

Abbreviations: RUM, radial, ulnar, median; RUMM, radial, ulnar, musculocutaneous, and median nerves.

It should also be noted that the analgesia produced by α_2-agonists is of a shorter duration than the sedation that is produced. Practitioners should be cognizant of this while assessing patient's pain status; sedation can potentially mask painful behaviors. Additionally, administration of an α_2-antagonist reverses the sedation and analgesia provided these drugs.

Although α_2-agonists should not be relied on as the sole analgesic agent, they can play a significant role in a balanced analgesic plan (**Table 6**). Doses administered at the time of premedication can act synergistically with opioids, improving analgesia and sedation while allowing lower doses of each drug to be used. Small doses given postoperatively can provide sedation and analgesia especially in animals experiencing dysphoria.

Further studies are needed, but α_2-agonists may be useful when used in a manner different from systemic administration. For example, they help as an adjuvant to local anesthetics in peripheral nerve blocks. One study in humans demonstrated that dexmedetomidine prolonged a peripheral nerve block performed with ropivacaine by approximately 60%.[34] Intra-articular injections of α_2-agonists also may be beneficial, as shown by studies involving humans undergoing arthroscopy[35] and rats suffering from arthritic pain.[36]

WOULD AN ANALGESIC ADJUNCT BE BENEFICIAL?

There are other classes of drugs that are not traditionally used in the management of perioperative pain but may be helpful as analgesic adjuncts especially when treating refractory pain states (**Table 7**). The drugs discussed here should be used in

Table 6
α_2-Agonists used for the treatment of acute pain in the dog and cat

Drug	Dosage in the Dog	Dosage in the Cat	Notes
Xylazine (Rompun SA)	0.1–0.5 mg/kg IM, IV	0.1–0.5 mg/kg IM, IV	Sedation, bradycardia, vomiting (especially in cats)
Dexmedetomidine (Dexdomitor)	0.005–0.02 mg/kg IM 0.001–0.005 mg/kg IV 0.001–0.003 mg/kg/h CRI	0.01–0.02 mg/kg IM 0.001–0.005 mg/kg IV 0.001–0.003 mg/kg/h CRI	Small doses useful in recovery period Even at low doses cardiovascular effects are significant
Clonidine (Catapres)	0.01 mg/kg IV 0.1 mg/15–20 kg transdermal patch	0.01 mg/kg IV	—
α_2-Antagonist			
Atipamezole (Antisedan)	0.05–0.2 mg/kg IV, IM Or 2–5 times the dexmedetomidine dose	0.05–0.2 mg/kg IV, IM Or 2–5 times the dexmedetomidine dose	IV administration usually reserved for emergency situations; this can cause excitement, delirium, and vomiting IM administration results in rapid and complete reversal of α_2-agonist effects, including analgesia

Abbreviations: CRI, constant rate infusion; IM, intramuscularly; IV, intravenously.

conjunction with known analgesics, such as opioids, because they may produce little analgesia when used alone. Additionally, caution should be used when administering some of these agents to veterinary patients. In some cases, little to no data are available regarding the efficacy of these drugs in acute pain states in dogs and cats. Extrapolation of human data should be done with prudence.

N-Methyl-D-Aspartate Antagonists

Ketamine is an *N*-methyl-D-aspartate receptor antagonist that may provide analgesia by binding to *N*-methyl-D-aspartate receptors and reducing central nervous system sensitization while increasing inhibitory nerve activity.[37] It seems that ketamine may be most effective when administered as a constant rate infusion before tissue injury.[38,39] Although analgesic doses are considerably smaller than anesthetic doses, side effects can be seen relating to sympathetic stimulation of the cardiovascular and nervous systems.

Anticonvulsants

Gabapentin may produce analgesia by reducing the release of neurotransmitters, such as substance P and glutamate, and interacting with γ-aminobutyric acid receptors in the spinal cord.[40] Additionally, gabapentin works synergistically with opioids to

Table 7
Analgesic adjuncts used for the treatment of acute pain in the dog and cat

Drug	Dosage in the Dog	Dosage in the Cat	Notes
Ketamine (Vetalar, Ketaset)	0.5 mg/kg IV 1.2 mg/kg/h IV CRI intraoperatively Can be reduced for recovery period	0.5 mg/kg IV 1.2 mg/kg/h IV CRI intraoperatively Can be reduced for recovery period	—
Gabapentin (Neurontin)	2.5–40 mg/kg PO q 8–12 h	5–10 mg/kg PO q 12 h	—
Amitriptyline (Elavil)	1–2 mg/kg PO q 12–24 h	5–10 mg/kg PO q 24 h	—
Duloxetine	Data unknown	Data unknown	—
Maropitant	1–5 mg/kg IV, SC 0.03–0.150 mg/kg/h IV CRI	—	No demonstrated analgesic effect in dogs or cats Reduces sevoflurane requirements in the dog
Trazodone	1.7–9.5 mg/kg PO q 8–24 h	—	No analgesic effect but may be useful in decreasing anxiety and facilitating postsurgical confinement

Abbreviations: CRI, constant rate infusion; IV, intravenously.

increase sedation and analgesia. Few studies have assessed the role of gabapentin in the perioperative period[40,41]; however, it may be useful in animals with neuropathic pain conditions. Side effects in dogs may include sleepiness and muscle weakness.

Tricyclic Antidepressants

This class of drugs is used extensively for the treatment of neuropathic pain in humans.[42] However, a recent review article evaluating the use of tricyclic antidepressants (TCAs) for the prevention of acute or chronic pain revealed therapeutic potential for TCAs, but evidence was lacking to support the clinical use of TCAs beyond controlled investigations.[43] One study exists demonstrating the effective use of amitriptyline for the treatment of neuropathic pain in dogs.[44] Therefore, the evidence supporting the use of TCAs in the management of acute pain in the dog is currently insufficient.

Serotonin–Norepinephrine Reuptake Inhibitor

Species-specific data relating to the efficacy of duloxetine (Cymbalta) in treating acute pain are lacking. A recent study in rats demonstrates that intrathecal or intraperitoneal administration does reduce hypersensitivity in a postoperative pain model,[45] and pharmacokinetic data of a single oral dose in the dog have been evaluated.[46] It should be noted that other analgesic drugs (some opioids, tramadol) also effect serotonin reuptake. Therefore, combinations of these drugs could result in serotonin toxicity.

Nonanalgesic Drugs

As discussed previously, emesis is a potential complication of opioid administration. The centrally acting antiemetic maropitant (Cerenia) blocks neurokinin-1 receptors in the chemoreceptor trigger zone and is labeled for use in the dog and cat. Although studies in other species (mice, rabbits) have demonstrated that neurokinin-1 antagonists induce analgesia, there are currently no studies demonstrating this in dogs or cats. Intravenous maropitant has been demonstrated to reduce sevoflurane requirements in the dog.[47] This should be considered when using maropitant before inhalant anesthesia and careful monitoring of anesthetic depth should be performed.

At times, postsurgical confinement is beneficial to promote healing and prevent damage to surgical repairs. The serotonin antagonist and reuptake inhibitor trazodone (Oleptro), used to facilitate this confinement in dogs after orthopedic surgery, was found to be efficacious and safe even when used in combination with other drugs, such as NSAIDs.[48]

WHAT NONPHARMACOLOGIC THERAPIES COULD BE INCORPORATED IN THE ANALGESIC PLAN?

Pharmacologic therapy will always form the basis of the analgesic plan, but the benefits of the most carefully planned analgesic protocol may not be realized unless additional aspects of perioperative care are addressed. This means incorporating minimally invasive surgery and gentle intraoperative handling of tissues, reducing stress in the patient with gentle handling, and optimizing fluid therapy. Additionally, appropriate nutrition should be included to aid in healing and recovery.

Cold therapy should be considered postoperatively because there is evidence that patients receiving cold compression therapy after orthopedic surgery exhibited decreased pain, swelling, and lameness during the first 24 hours after surgery.[49] Acupuncture and electroacupuncture may also reduce the need for systemic analgesics postoperatively.[50] Low-level laser therapy may also shorten the time to return to function.[51]

SUMMARY

Untreated or undermanaged perioperative pain has systemic effects that may negatively impact a patient's welfare and return to function. A consistent plan that assesses a patient's pain and comfort at regular intervals during the perioperative period should be incorporated into practice. Validated pain assessment tools are available for use in dogs and cats. Multimodal analgesic plans should be created for individual patients and modified according to pain assessments. These plans, based on a thorough history, physical examination, and knowledge of the expected pain, should usually be combinations of an opioid, an NSAID, a local anesthetic, and nonpharmacologic analgesic techniques. Analgesic adjuncts and α_2-agonists should be considered and added to the protocol as needed. It should always be remembered that the gold standard of pain assessment is response to analgesic therapy. If in doubt, administer analgesics.

REFERENCES

1. Wiese AJ, Yaksh TL. Chapter 2 - Nociception and pain mechanisms. In: Gaynor JS, Muir WW, editors. Handbook of veterinary pain management. 3rd edition. St. Louis (MO): Mosby; 2015. p. 10–41.

2. Wiese AJ. Chapter 5 - Assessing pain: pain behaviors. In: Gaynor JS, Muir WW, editors. Handbook of veterinary pain management. 3rd edition. St. Louis (MO): Mosby; 2015. p. 67–97.

3. Lamont LA. Feline perioperative pain management. Vet Clin North Am Small Anim Pract 2002;32(4):747–63, v.

4. Mathews K, Kronen PW, Lascelles D, et al. Guidelines for recognition, assessment and treatment of pain: WSAVA Global Pain Council members and co-authors of this document. J Small Anim Pract 2014;55(6):E10–68.

5. Ong CK, Lirk P, Seymour RA, et al. The efficacy of preemptive analgesia for acute postoperative pain management: a meta-analysis. Anesth Analg 2005;100(3): 757–73 table of contents.

6. Bufalari A, Maggio C, Cerasoli I, et al. Preemptive carprofen for peri-operative analgesia in dogs undergoing Tibial Plateau Leveling Osteotomy (TPLO): a prospective, randomized, blinded, placebo controlled clinical trial. Schweiz Arch Tierheilkd 2012;154(3):105–11.

7. Nakagawa K, Miyagawa Y, Takemura N, et al. Influence of preemptive analgesia with meloxicam before resection of the unilateral mammary gland on postoperative cardiovascular parameters in dogs. J Vet Med Sci 2007;69(9):939–44.

8. Troncy E, Junot S, Keroack S, et al. Results of preemptive epidural administration of morphine with or without bupivacaine in dogs and cats undergoing surgery: 265 cases (1997-1999). J Am Vet Med Assoc 2002;221(5):666–72.

9. Elanco. Elanco product website. Available at: http://www.elancovet.com/products/recuvyra/?AspxAutoDetectCookieSupport=1. Accessed February 28, 2015.

10. Freise KJ, Newbound GC, Tudan C, et al. Pharmacokinetics and the effect of application site on a novel, long-acting transdermal fentanyl solution in healthy laboratory Beagles. J Vet Pharmacol Ther 2012;35(Suppl 2):27–33.

11. Linton DD, Wilson MG, Newbound GC, et al. The effectiveness of a long-acting transdermal fentanyl solution compared to buprenorphine for the control of postoperative pain in dogs in a randomized, multicentered clinical study. J Vet Pharmacol Ther 2012;35(Suppl 2):53–64.

12. Martinez SA, Wilson MG, Linton DD, et al. The safety and effectiveness of a long-acting transdermal fentanyl solution compared with oxymorphone for the control of postoperative pain in dogs: a randomized, multicentered clinical study. J Vet Pharmacol Ther 2014;37(4):394–405.

13. Freise KJ, Newbound GC, Tudan C, et al. Naloxone reversal of an overdose of a novel, long-acting transdermal fentanyl solution in laboratory Beagles. J Vet Pharmacol Ther 2012;35(Suppl 2):45–51.

14. Steagall PV, Monteiro-Steagall BP, Taylor PM. A review of the studies using buprenorphine in cats. J Vet Intern Med 2014;28(3):762–70.

15. Abbott. Available at: http://www.abbottanimalhealth.com/docs/SIM-2013.pdf. Accessed October 15, 2014.

16. Ide S, Minami M, Ishihara K, et al. Mu opioid receptor-dependent and independent components in effects of tramadol. Neuropharmacology 2006;51(3): 651–8.

17. Kongara K, Chambers JP, Johnson CB. Effects of tramadol, morphine or their combination in dogs undergoing ovariohysterectomy on peri-operative electroencephalographic responses and post-operative pain. N Z Vet J 2012;60(2):129–35.

18. Teixeira RC, Monteiro ER, Campagnol D, et al. Effects of tramadol alone, in combination with meloxicam or dipyrone, on postoperative pain and the analgesic requirement in dogs undergoing unilateral mastectomy with or without ovariohysterectomy. Vet Anaesth Analg 2013;40(6):641–9.

19. Brondani JT, Loureiro Luna SP, Beier SL, et al. Analgesic efficacy of perioperative use of vedaprofen, tramadol or their combination in cats undergoing ovariohysterectomy. J Feline Med Surg 2009;11(6):420–9.
20. Pypendop BH, Siao KT, Ilkiw JE. Effects of tramadol hydrochloride on the thermal threshold in cats. Am J Vet Res 2009;70(12):1465–70.
21. Mercadante S, Porzio G, Gebbia V. New opioids. J Clin Oncol 2014;32(16): 1671–6.
22. Kogel B, Terlinden R, Schneider J. Characterisation of tramadol, morphine and tapentadol in an acute pain model in Beagle dogs. Vet Anaesth Analg 2014; 41(3):297–304.
23. Livingston A. Mechanism of action of nonsteroidal anti-inflammatory drugs. Vet Clin North Am Small Anim Pract 2000;30(4):773–81, vi.
24. Vanegas H, Schaible HG. Prostaglandins and cyclooxygenases [correction of cyclooxygenases] in the spinal cord. Prog Neurobiol 2001;64(4):327–63.
25. Luna SP, Basilio AC, Steagall PV, et al. Evaluation of adverse effects of long-term oral administration of carprofen, etodolac, flunixin meglumine, ketoprofen, and meloxicam in dogs. Am J Vet Res 2007;68(3):258–64.
26. Elwood C, Boswood A, Simpson K, et al. Renal failure after flunixin meglumine administration. Vet Rec 1992;130(26):582–3.
27. MacPhail CM, Lappin MR, Meyer DJ, et al. Hepatocellular toxicosis associated with administration of carprofen in 21 dogs. J Am Vet Med Assoc 1998; 212(12):1895–901.
28. Epstein M, Rodan I, Griffenhagen G, et al. 2015 AAHA/AAFP pain management guidelines for dogs and cats. J Am Anim Hosp Assoc 2015;51(2): 67–84.
29. Butterworth JF 4th, Strichartz GR. Molecular mechanisms of local anesthesia: a review. Anesthesiology 1990;72(4):711–34.
30. Liu PL, Feldman HS, Giasi R, et al. Comparative CNS toxicity of lidocaine, etidocaine, bupivacaine, and tetracaine in awake dogs following rapid intravenous administration. Anesth Analg 1983;62(4):375–9.
31. Moller RA, Covino BG. Cardiac electrophysiologic effects of lidocaine and bupivacaine. Anesth Analg 1988;67(2):107–14.
32. Pypendop BH, Verstegen JP. Hemodynamic effects of medetomidine in the dog: a dose titration study. Vet Surg 1998;27(6):612–22.
33. Klide AM, Calderwood HW, Soma LR. Cardiopulmonary effects of xylazine in dogs. Am J Vet Res 1975;36(7):931–5.
34. Marhofer D, Kettner SC, Marhofer P, et al. Dexmedetomidine as an adjuvant to ropivacaine prolongs peripheral nerve block: a volunteer study. Br J Anaesth 2013;110(3):438–42.
35. Joshi W, Reuben SS, Kilaru PR, et al. Postoperative analgesia for outpatient arthroscopic knee surgery with intraarticular clonidine and/or morphine. Anesth Analg 2000;90(5):1102–6.
36. Ansah OB, Pertovaara A. Peripheral suppression of arthritic pain by intraarticular fadolmidine, an alpha 2-adrenoceptor agonist, in the rat. Anesth Analg 2007; 105(1):245–50.
37. Felsby S, Nielsen J, Arendt-Nielsen L, et al. NMDA receptor blockade in chronic neuropathic pain: a comparison of ketamine and magnesium chloride. Pain 1996; 64(2):283–91.
38. Hamilton SM, Johnston SA, Broadstone RV. Evaluation of analgesia provided by the administration of epidural ketamine in dogs with a chemically induced synovitis. Vet Anaesth Analg 2005;32(1):30–9.

39. Wagner AE, Walton JA, Hellyer PW, et al. Use of low doses of ketamine administered by constant rate infusion as an adjunct for postoperative analgesia in dogs. J Am Vet Med Assoc 2002;221(1):72–5.
40. Takeuchi Y, Takasu K, Honda M, et al. Neurochemical evidence that supraspinally administered gabapentin activates the descending noradrenergic system after peripheral nerve injury. Eur J Pharmacol 2007;556(1–3):69–74.
41. Wagner AE, Mich PM, Uhrig SR, et al. Clinical evaluation of perioperative administration of gabapentin as an adjunct for postoperative analgesia in dogs undergoing amputation of a forelimb. J Am Vet Med Assoc 2010;236(7):751–6.
42. Sindrup SH, Otto M, Finnerup NB, et al. Antidepressants in the treatment of neuropathic pain. Basic Clin Pharmacol Toxicol 2005;96(6):399–409.
43. Wong K, Phelan R, Kalso E, et al. Antidepressant drugs for prevention of acute and chronic postsurgical pain: early evidence and recommended future directions. Anesthesiology 2014;121(3):591–608.
44. Cashmore RG, Harcourt-Brown TR, Freeman PM, et al. Clinical diagnosis and treatment of suspected neuropathic pain in three dogs. Aust Vet J 2009;87(1):45–50.
45. Sun YH, Li HS, Zhu C, et al. The analgesia effect of duloxetine on post-operative pain via intrathecal or intraperitoneal administration. Neurosci Lett 2014;568:6–11.
46. Baek IH, Lee BY, Kang W, et al. Pharmacokinetic analysis of two different doses of duloxetine following oral administration in dogs. Drug Res 2013;63(8):404–8.
47. Alvillar BM, Boscan P, Mama KR, et al. Effect of epidural and intravenous use of the neurokinin-1 (NK-1) receptor antagonist maropitant on the sevoflurane minimum alveolar concentration (MAC) in dogs. Vet Anaesth Analg 2012;39(2):201–5.
48. Gruen ME, Roe SC, Griffith E, et al. Use of trazodone to facilitate postsurgical confinement in dogs. J Am Vet Med Assoc 2014;245(3):296–301.
49. Drygas KA, McClure SR, Goring RL, et al. Effect of cold compression therapy on postoperative pain, swelling, range of motion, and lameness after tibial plateau leveling osteotomy in dogs. J Am Vet Med Assoc 2011;238(10):1284–91.
50. Groppetti D, Pecile AM, Sacerdote P, et al. Effectiveness of electroacupuncture analgesia compared with opioid administration in a dog model: a pilot study. Br J Anaesth 2011;107(4):612–8.
51. Draper WE, Schubert TA, Clemmons RM, et al. Low-level laser therapy reduces time to ambulation in dogs after hemilaminectomy: a preliminary study. J Small Anim Pract 2012;53(8):465–9.
52. Pypendop BH, Ilkiw JE. Assessment of the hemodynamic effects of lidocaine administered IV in isoflurane-anesthetized cats. Am J Vet Res 2005;66(4):661–8.
53. Portela DA, Romano M, Briganti A. Retrospective clinical evaluation of ultrasound guided transverse abdominis plane block in dogs undergoing mastectomy. Vet Anaesth Analg 2014;41(3):319–24.
54. Abelson AL, McCobb EC, Shaw S, et al. Use of wound soaker catheters for the administration of local anesthetic for post-operative analgesia: 56 cases. Vet Anaesth Analg 2009;36(6):597–602.

Nursing Care

Care of the Perioperative Patient

Harold Davis, BA, RVT, VTS (ECC) (Anesth)

KEYWORDS

- Nursing process • Artificial airway management • Coupage • Catheter

KEY POINTS

- The veterinary technician must have an understanding and working knowledge of a variety of nursing care techniques.
- The technician should know what it takes to perform the technique and be aware of risk factors and potential complications and what action is to be taken if the complication is encountered.
- As a part of nursing care, technicians should constantly evaluate the patient's condition and ask if the nursing goals are being met and if risk factors are turning into complications.
- It is better to be proactive rather than reactive to potential complications.

INTRODUCTION

Although the veterinarian is responsible for making the diagnosis, discussing prognosis with the owners, performing surgery, and prescribing medication and therapy, the veterinary technician is charged with providing the nursing care. To provide nursing care, the veterinary technician must be knowledgeable and skilled in patient assessment and patient care techniques. The veterinary technician should also be knowledgeable in potential risk factors/complications; this puts the veterinary technician in a position of being proactive rather than reactive to problems. This article reviews nursing care as it pertains to the various body systems and addresses some common risk factors and complications.

DEVELOPING NURSING CARE PLANS

Nursing care plans are developed to meet patient care needs based on the disease processes. The ultimate goal is to enhance the delivery of patient care. There are a variety of ways to develop nursing care plans. The nursing process is a problem-solving

The author has nothing to disclose.
William R. Pritchard Veterinary Medical Teaching Hospital, University of California, Davis, One Shields Avenue, Davis, CA 95616, USA
E-mail address: hhdavis@ucdavis.edu

approach used in the development of a plan of care for each patient. In the case of the veterinary patient, a plan of care is a list of the interventions the technician intends to initiate to restore the animal to a state of well-being.[1] In human nursing, the nursing process comprises 5 phases or components: assessment, nursing diagnosis, planning, implementation, and evaluation. Veterinary technicians are not allowed to diagnose; therefore, the authors rename the nursing diagnosis the technician's conclusion.

Assessment

The purpose of assessment is to help identify the patient's problems or condition. Patient assessment is the data collection and analysis portion of the nursing process. The basic categories of techniques used in the assessment include interaction, observation, and measurement. Data may come from a variety of sources: owners provide a history, members of the health care team share information concerning the patient, the technician or veterinarian performs a physical examination, review of previous medical history and laboratory data, and collection of physiologic parameters (eg, blood pressure, electrocardiography [ECG], heart rate, temperature, central venous pressure).

Technician Conclusion (Analysis)

In human nursing, the next step is arriving at the nursing diagnosis. The nursing diagnosis is based on the patient assessment and is a label that conveniently describes in a few words what the problem is. The North American Nursing Diagnosis Association (NANDA) developed a list of approved nursing diagnoses. A similar approved list does not formally exist for veterinary technicians. However, Rockett and colleagues[2] provide a list of technician evaluations (**Box 1**) that might be considered analogues to the NANDA nursing diagnosis. The technician evaluation is the veterinary technician's conclusion about the animal's or owner's response to physical and psychological challenges and is based on the data collected during the assessment.

Following the assessment, the veterinary technician analyzes the data obtained in the assessment phase. The technician tries to cluster or group those abnormalities that fit together and help identify a problem. Clustering the signs helps to organize information in a systematic manner and facilitate the formation of the technician's conclusions. Ultimately, the technician's conclusions serve as an aid in determining proper nursing interventions.

The veterinary technician should think about what it takes to meet desired goals and potential risk factors/complications. The veterinary technician should also be aware of how to recognize the risk factors/complications and what actions are taken to correct any problems. In arriving at the technician's conclusions the veterinary technician is not trying to make a diagnosis but rather working with the veterinarian to help provide the best care for the patient. The technician can make a judgment about the patient's response. For example, the veterinarian might ultimately diagnose pneumothorax and hypovolemic shock because the veterinary technician made an assessment of altered ventilation/gas exchange and poor perfusion. Based on the technician conclusion, the veterinary technician could begin to anticipate the needs of the patient and veterinarian and prepare for the appropriate intervention.

Planning Care

The ability to select appropriate interventions should follow naturally from the identification of the technician conclusions. The following questions may be helpful to the veterinary technician in developing nursing care plans:

1. What are the goals of therapy?

Box 1
A list of technician evaluations

Abnormal eating behavior

Acute pain

Aggression

Altered gas diffusion

Altered mentation

Altered oral health

Altered sensory perception

Altered urinary production

Altered ventilation

Anxiety

Bowel incontinence

Cardiac insufficiency

Chronic pain

Client coping deficit

Client knowledge deficit

Constipation

Decreased perfusion

Diarrhea

Electrolyte imbalance

Exercise intolerance

Fear

Hyperthermia

Hypervolemia

Hypothermia

Hypovolemia

Impaired tissue integrity

Inappropriate elimination

Ineffective nursing

Noncompliant nursing

Obstructed airway

Overweight

Postoperative compliance

Preoperative compliance

Reduced mobility

Reproductive dysfunction

Risk of aspiration

Risk of infection

Risk of infection transmission

Self-care deficit

Self-inflicted injury

Sleep disturbance

Status within appropriate limits

Underweight

Urinary incontinence

Vomiting/nausea

Adapted from Rockett J, Lattanzio C, Anderson K. Technician evaluations with suggested interventions. Patient assessment, intervention and documentation for the veterinary technician. New York: Delmar Cengage Learning; 2009. p. 57; with permission.

2. What adverse effects could the disease have on the patient and how would it be recognized?
3. What action would be taken if the patient developed the problem?
4. What drugs are being administered to the patient; what adverse effects can the drugs cause; and how would one recognize the drug reaction?
5. What type of monitoring is generally used for the given disease process?
6. What type of general nursing care is required, that is, intravenous (IV) catheter care, urinary catheter care, and/or recumbent patient care?

Part of the planning process includes consideration of general nursing care procedures. It is helpful to have a checklist of daily nursing care tasks (**Fig. 1**). Standing orders could be made for certain nursing care tasks; these tasks are always performed on a patient unless otherwise directed by the veterinarian.

Implementation

In this phase, the clinician's orders are carried out and the nursing plan is put into action.

Evaluation

Evaluation is the final phase, although it may occur throughout the nursing process. During the evaluation phase, the veterinary technician is looking to see if therapy is improving the patient's condition. If the patient is not meeting the desired goals, the question "Why not?" should be asked. There are several issues to consider: (1) maybe it is too soon to evaluate, (2) perhaps the intervention should be intensified, (3) there may be some other factor that has not been considered, and (4) the nursing evaluation could be incorrect. If the patient's condition does not improve or it worsens, the veterinarian must be notified and a new plan needs to be developed.

RESPIRATORY NURSING CARE
Artificial Airway Management

Artificial airways include tracheostomy and endotracheal tubes; they are used to maintain a patient airway and in some cases facilitate mechanical ventilation (see Oxygenation and Ventilation by Rozanski elsewhere in this issue for discussion of mechanical ventilation.) The principles of artificial airway management entail airway humidification, tracheal suctioning, coupage, tracheostomy site care, and oral care.

Daily Patient Care Checklist

Beginning of shift checklist

Review cases (record and orders)	[ ]
Conduct rounds	[ ]
Check all catheters and monitoring devices	[ ]
Check emergency equipment	[ ]
Organize the "to do list"	[ ]

Patient care check list

Evaluate patient status (mentation, TPR, auscultation)	[ ]
Weigh and record (acute or gradual change?)	[ ]
Is the patient urinating? (Palpate bladder if not)	[ ]
Is the patient eating and drinking?	[ ]
a) Is it consuming enough calories?	[ ]
b) Is it consuming enough water?	[ ]
Are the psychological needs being met? (Walks, TLC)	[ ]
Wound and/or bandage care as ordered	[ ]
Is the patient clean and comfortable?	[ ]
Are steps being taken to prevent nosocomial infection?	[ ]
Are steps being taken to control pain?	[ ]

Nonambulatory patient care

Turn the patient q 2–4 h	[ ]
Is the cage/run well padded?	[ ]
Check for decubital ulcer formation	[ ]
Are there any contraindications to physical therapy?	[ ]
Consider risk factors for recumbent patients	[ ]

Catheters

Perform IV catheter care q 48 h or PRN	[ ]
Flush capped IV catheter with saline or heparinized saline q 4 h or perform heparin lock q 12 h	[ ]
Urinary catheter care q 8 h	[ ]
Chest drain/feeding tube care q 24 h	[ ]
Change IV administration sets q 96 h	[ ]
Artificial airway management/care q 4 h or PRN	[ ]

Fig. 1. Daily patient care checklist for general nursing care. PRN, as needed; TLC, tender loving care; TPR, temperature, pulse and respiration.

Humidification

Normally, when the animal breathes, the inhaled air is humidified through the nasal passages. Because the tracheostomy and endotracheal tube bypasses this, the animal is unable to humidify the air that it breathes. Therefore, some source of humidification must be provided for the patient.

Humidification can be done continuously or intermittently. Humidification is performed with a jet or ultrasonic nebulizer and usually takes 15 to 20 minutes. Sterile water is added to the nebulizer canister. Jet nebulizers are attached to an oxygen source and form saline particles by passing a high-velocity gas stream across the top of a capillary tube that is immersed in saline. The saline is drawn up into the tube and broken into particles, with the larger particles dropping out of the gas stream. Smaller droplets are delivered to the patient. Particle size ranges between 0.5 and 30 μm. Ultrasonic nebulizers are electrically driven units that convert electric energy into high-frequency vibrations that are transmitted to the nebulizer reservoir. A fine, dense, cool fog with a particle size less than 5 μm in diameter is produced. The nebulizer can be attached to a cage or incubator, thereby nebulizing the enclosed environment (**Fig. 2**) or held in close proximity to the end of the tracheostomy or endotracheal tube.

Coupage

After nebulization and before suctioning, the patient should be coupaged if there are no contraindications such as coagulation defects and thoracic wall injury. Coupage is used to loosen secretions and facilitate airway clearance. Using cupped hands, the thorax is rhythmically patted for 5 minutes. The vibration of the chest should loosen secretions facilitating airway suctioning. Coupage should not be done if it is stressful to the patient.

Suctioning

Tracheal suctioning is important for the removal of secretions from airways. Respiratory secretions are continually produced and accumulated as a result of poor function of the mucociliary elevator. Patients with an artificial airway cannot cough and clear their airway.

Tracheal suctioning should be performed approximately every 4 hours, with the frequency adjusted depending on the volume of secretions the patient is producing. Both tracheostomy and endotracheal tubes may require suctioning.

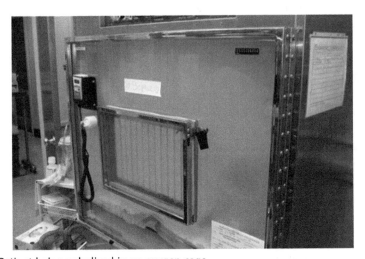

Fig. 2. Patient being nebulized in an oxygen cage.

The technique for suctioning a tracheostomy tube and endotracheal tube are essentially the same. However, with the tracheostomy tubes that use inner cannulas, the inner cannula can be removed when it is time to suction the airway and placed in a 1:1 dilution of sterile water and hydrogen peroxide. For suctioning, the following supplies are needed: (1) suction catheter, (2) suction source, (3) sterile gloves, (4) container with sterile water, and (5) oxygen source.

Open suction catheters such as the Triflo suction catheter (Cardinal Health, Dublin, OH, USA) are commonly used to suction airways in ventilated and nonventilated patients. Sterile gloves must be worn when using this type of suction catheter. The Ballard-style suction catheter (Halyard Health, formerly Kimberley-Clark, Alpharetta, GA, USA) can be used with patients on ventilator. The Ballard catheter is a closed-system catheter (**Fig. 3**), which means the catheter is actually enclosed in a protective plastic sleeve and does not require the use of sterile gloves. The catheter may remain attached to the patient and ventilator system if desired. A suction catheter that is 50% of the inner diameter of the internal tracheostomy or endotracheal tube is used. To determine the appropriate French size of the catheter, the internal tracheostomy tube size is divided by 2 and this number is multiplied by 3.[3]

If the patient is on mechanical ventilation, before suctioning the patient should be placed on 100% oxygen for a few minutes to protect against hypoxemia during suctioning. The catheter is passed down the tracheostomy or endotracheal tube without suction. With a tracheostomy tube, the catheter is passed about 2 cm beyond the end of the tube. With an endotracheal tube, it is passed until resistance is met. The

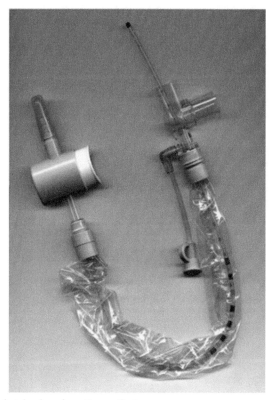

Fig. 3. The Ballard-style closed suction catheter.

catheter is backed out a few millimeters and the finger is placed over the vent hole on the open suction catheter or thumb button on the Ballard-style catheter. The catheter is backed out using a twirling motion suctioning for no longer than 10 seconds. The secretions should be evaluated and characterized and the procedure repeated until no further secretions are obtained or the secretions become clear.

Tracheal suctioning should always result in some airway secretions. If not, it is not because they are not there, it is because they are too dry. Better airway humidification and secretion liquefaction is needed. Systemic hydration is also a major contributor.

Tracheostomy site care
If the patient has a tracheostomy, tracheostomy site care should be performed several times daily. A dressing (bib, **Fig. 4**) is applied to promote skin integrity and help prevent infection at the site of the stoma/insertion site. Tracheal secretions can cause maceration and excoriation at the stoma site. The protective bib is removed and the site inspected for signs of inflammation, infection, or skin breakdown from pressure exerted by the flange. The area should be cleaned with sterile cotton-tip applicators or gauze squares and normal saline every 8 hours and the bib replaced.

Endotracheal tube care
Endotracheal tube cuff pressure should be checked every 4 hours. There are no specific standards for changing endotracheal tubes at regular intervals.

Oral care
Oral care is performed to minimize the risk of ventilator-associated pneumonia. In the intubated patient it is important to make sure the tongue is not draped out over the teeth, endotracheal tube, or mouth speculum. The tongue should not be incorporated into the endotracheal tube tie. If in use, the pulse oximeter probe should be moved to a new location every 2 hours.

1. Gently suction the mouth and pharynx every 4 hours.
2. Then wipe the gums, teeth, tongue, and mucous membranes with chlorhexidine mouth wash solution.
3. Moisten the tongue with water and place it comfortably back within the mouth.

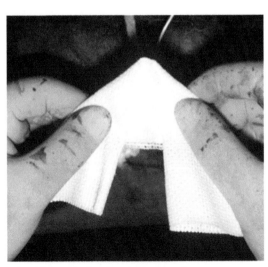

Fig. 4. Making a tracheal bib out of a 4 × 4 gauze pad.

Complications

A variety of complications can occur with artificial airways and suctioning. Artificial airway complications include the following:

1. Airway obstruction from mucous or dried tracheal secretions (**Fig. 5**)
2. Infection of the tracheal stoma/insertion site
3. Tracheal necrosis, stenosis, and erosion as a result of excessive pressure exerted on the tracheal wall by the cuff or tube itself

   Tracheal-related suctioning complications include the following:

1. Suction catheter–related trauma
2. Vasovagal stimulation resulting in collapse and bradycardia
3. Arrhythmias
4. Hypoxemia secondary to atelectasis
5. Small airway collapse secondary to suctioning

Chest Tubes

Chest tubes are used to evacuate the pleural cavity of fluid or air. Evacuation of the pleural cavity can be either intermittent or continuous.

When chest tubes are inserted, they should be secured with a purse string around the tube at the site of entry and a finger trap suture pattern. The chest tube is connected to a Christmas tree female Luer connector and 3-way stopcock with a Luer lock if intermittent aspirations are going to be performed (**Fig. 6**). If continuous suction is to be used, the chest tube is connected directly to the chest drainage system via a double Christmas tree connector. A pinch and slide clamp may be used as added protection to maintain a closed system if not attached to continuous drainage. The chest tube may be marked with indelible ink as it exits the skin so the tube can be observed for tube migration. The insertion site is covered with a sterile gauze pad. A light bandage may be placed around the thorax or a stockinette.

Chest tube care

The goal of chest tube care is to minimize or prevent chest tube–related complications. Chest tube care is performed every 24 hours. Care of the chest tube entails bandage removal, inspection, cleaning, and rebandaging. Following bandage removal, the chest tube site is inspected, looking for signs of infection (erythema, swelling, heat, and purulent discharge). In addition, the chest tube is inspected for tube migration and subcutaneous emphysema. Following inspection, the site is

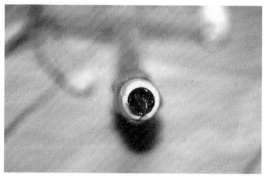

Fig. 5. A tracheostomy tube with a dried mucous plug.

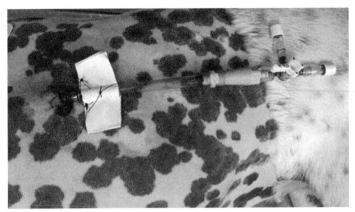

Fig. 6. Chest tube insertion site; note the finger trap suture pattern and the Christmas tree Luer connector and 3-way stopcock.

cleaned with an antimicrobial scrub and solution. The chest tube site is re-dressed. A swab from a chest drain site should be considered if clinical signs of infection are present. All findings during chest tube care should be documented in the medical record.

Chest Drainage

Intermittent (manual) aspiration

Intermittent or manual aspiration of the chest tube is usually carried out via a 3-way stopcock and large syringe at specified intervals. Strict attention to aseptic technique must be followed when handling the chest tube. The force of aspiration should be mild, because extremely low subatmospheric pressures can be easily generated and can be damaging to thoracic tissues. The chest tube is aspirated until negative pressure is achieved. Repositioning the patient and aspirating the chest tube may facilitate the additional collection of fluid or air. Documentation of the volume of air or fluid and the gross appearance of the fluid is made in the patient record. Any chest fluid aspirated is considered an abnormal fluid loss, which is included in the patient's fluid therapy plan.

CONTINUOUS SUCTION/ASPIRATION

If continuous chest drainage is required, the patient is attached to a system with a water seal, such as a 3-chamber disposable chest drainage system. The 3 chambers are the collection, underwater seal, and suction control chambers. The collection chamber allows for collection and quantitation of fluid or cellular debris that is evacuated from the pleural cavity. The underwater seal maintains a closed system or isolates the patient so that the suction may be disconnected without exposing the pleural space to air. If the patient has a pneumothorax or there is a leak in the system, bubbling is seen in the underwater seal. The third chamber is the suction control chamber. It controls the amount of suction that is being generated at the end of the chest tube in the pleural space. The amount of suction is determined by the amount of water in the suction control chamber. If water is poured into the chamber to the 15 cm mark, that is equivalent to 15 cm of negative or subatmospheric pressure. The amount of suction for an individual patient depends on what is being evacuated. As a general guideline, a range of 10 to 15 cm H_2O is used if air is being evacuated; if it is viscous fluid or debris, then a range of 15 to 20 cm H_2O is used.[4,5]

NURSING CONSIDERATIONS

The following are general nursing management guidelines:

1. Chest drainage systems require 24 hour nursing supervision.
2. Maintain sterility while setting up the system.
3. Maintain the system and tubing at or ideally below the level of the patient and upright.
4. Dependent loops containing fluid can completely block fluid drainage within 30 minutes and change pleural pressures from -18 cm H_2O to $+8$ cm H_2O, a change of 26 cm H_2O in pressure. If a dependent loop cannot be avoided, lifting and draining it every 15 minutes maintains adequate drainage.[6,7]
5. Document the amount of suction used.
6. Note presence or absence of bubbling in the underwater seal; record the number of bubbles/minute each hour. If bubbles appear continuously, then assess for leaks in the system (**Table 1**).
7. Mark the drainage level outside of the collection chamber every 4 to 8 hours or as ordered by the clinician.
8. Document the character of the drainage.
9. Check the patient's respiratory status and mucous membrane color at regular intervals as dictated by the patient's condition.
10. Check the condition of the chest tube insertion site, and perform chest tube care at least every 24 hours.
11. Monitor for equipment failure.
12. Keep 2 chest tube clamps with the patient in the event of inadvertent disconnection.

Table 1
Steps to troubleshoot a continuous closed chest drainage system

Problem	Cause	Solution
Constant bubbling in the underwater seal	1. Air leak in the chest 2. Leak around the chest tube insertion site 3. Leak in the drainage system	1. To isolate the leak, at the insertion site, occlude the chest tube or drainage tubing for a moment (<1 min); observe for bubbles. If no bubbles, the air is being produced by the patient. If bubbles continue, then there is a leak in the system. Progressing toward the chest drain, repeat the occlusion and observation 2. Reapply the occlusive dressing 3. Assess and tighten all connections
Nothing is being removed despite evidence of air in the pleural space	1. Chest tube is clamped 2. Tube obstruction with debris 3. Kinked tubing 4. Suction control chamber water level is low	1. Remove the clamp 2. Milk the tubing: starting at the proximal end, gently squeeze and release along its length. This is not to be confused with stripping the chest tube (squeezing the length of tubing without release) Consider flushing the chest tube with a small amount of 0.9% NaCl 3. Check tubing for kinks (palpate the subcutaneous tissue as well) 4. Check and refill water level in the suction control chamber to the appropriate level

13. The chest tube is removed when the underlying disease process has resolved. Some fluid is expected as a normal response to the presence of the chest tube. The normal amount of fluid generated by the presence of the chest tube may range up to 0.5 to 2.0 mL/kg/d.

CARDIOVASCULAR NURSING CARE
Cardiovascular Monitoring Techniques

Arterial blood pressure and continuous electrocardiographic monitoring

Arterial blood pressure is measured by indirect and direct methods. Arterial blood pressure is the product of cardiac output and systemic vascular resistance. Blood pressure monitoring has become more common in clinical practice. The American College of Veterinary Anesthesiologist and Analgesia recommends blood pressure monitoring during anesthesia for all patients with moderate to severe systemic disease.[8,9] See Perioperative Blood Pressure Control and Management by Duke-Novakovski and Carr elsewhere in this issue for further discussion of blood pressure and Perioperative Monitoring of Heart Rate and Rhythm by Oyama for a discussion of ECGs.

Vascular Catheter Care and Maintenance

Intravascular catheter maintenance

IV catheter care should be performed every 48 hours or on an as-needed basis if the site gets soiled. The catheter dressing should be removed and the site inspected. The site should be examined for any signs of phlebitis, infection, and thrombosis, and, if present, the catheter should be removed. The catheter should be aspirated and flushed to establish the patency of the catheter. While flushing the catheter with saline or heparinized saline, the insertion site should be observed for fluid leakage or pain during injection. If either is observed, the catheter should be removed.

If any portion of the catheter is exposed, this should be recorded in the medical record, and the catheter should not be reinserted. If the catheter site looks good, the site should be cleaned with chlorhexidine solution. When the catheter site is dry, a sterile 2 × 2 gauze pad is placed over it and the bandage reapplied. It is no longer recommended to place antibiotic ointment at catheter insertion sites.[10] Catheter care findings are documented in the patient's medical record.

IV catheters should be replaced only when clinically indicated, and routine replacement every 72 to 96 hours is not necessary. As long as routine catheter care is performed, and the catheter removed when problems are first noticed, one can often exceed the 72-hour rule. A study of peripheral and jugular venous catheter contamination in dogs and cats supports this.[11]

IV catheters should be observed several times a day. If the catheter bandage is wet, the reason should be identified and the bandage should be changed. Swelling distal to the catheter may indicate an excessively tight bandage or tape. Swelling proximal to the catheter may be due to fluid infiltration.

The human literature suggests that normal saline (without heparin) may be as effective as heparinized saline in the maintenance of catheter patency.[12,13] In one veterinary study, flushes of 0.9% sodium chloride were found to be as effective as 10 IU/mL heparinized saline flushes in maintaining patency of 18-Ga peripheral venous catheters in dogs for up to 42 hours. The investigators suggested that heparinized flushes may be warranted in peripheral catheters placed with the intention of performing serial blood draws.[14]

All unused ports on catheters should be flushed regularly with saline or heparinized saline to maintain catheter patency. The author uses 4 U/mL of heparinized saline (1000 U/250 mL normal saline) every 4 hours. Bags of heparinized saline should be discarded every 12 to 24 hours to minimize the risk of contamination. If a catheter port is not going to be used for a prolonged period, an alternative is to use a heparin lock. The dead space of the catheter is filled with 100 U/mL heparin every 12 hours. The concentrated heparin solution is never flushed into the patient; instead, it is aspirated before administering medications or before replacing the heparin lock. Clear labeling of such ports to avoid inadvertent flushing of the concentrated heparin into the patient is important.

Arterial catheter maintenance
The arterial catheter is either attached to a continuous flush system or flushed with heparinized saline every 2 hours. The toes should be checked for warmth every 2 to 4 hours. If the toes are cool, the catheter should be removed. This care is especially important in cats, as they have poor collateral circulation and run the risk of losing toes. Catheter care similar to venous catheter care is performed every 48 hours. Fluids and drugs are not administered via the artery because of the potential risk of vascular damage and subsequent tissue necrosis. Complications include hemorrhage and infection.

Constant rate infusions
Many analgesics and cardiac or vasoactive drugs are administered as constant rate infusions (CRIs) via syringe pump or fluid infusion pump. With regard to analgesics, the main advantage of a CRI is that it avoids peaks and valleys that are typically seen with opioid bolus dosing. In addition, a lower dose of the drug may be administered over time. Cardiac and vasoactive drugs have a rapid onset of action and a short elimination half-life and must be administered as a CRI to maintain constant serum concentrations.

One must be able to set up, administer, and monitor the effects of the CRI. Spreadsheets can be made to calculate drug dilutions for commonly used infusions; this helps to minimize calculation errors.

There are a few simple formulas that can be used to calculate CRIs. A dosing scheme of micrograms per kilogram per minute is used for many drugs.

Formula 1: Drug dosage (micrograms per kilogram per minute) × body weight (kilograms) = Weight in milligrams to be added to a solution for a total volume of 250 mL. The CRI is given at a rate of 15 mL/h. The final volume and infusion rate remain constant. If 15 mL/h is too large a volume, one can double the concentration and half the rate.

Formula 2: The following formula solves for the weight of drug in milligrams (M) to be added to a base solution.

$$M = (D)\ (W)\ (V)/(R)\ (16.67)$$

The following formula solves for the rate (R) if dosage is adjusted.

$$R = (D\ \text{adjusted})\ (W)\ (V)/(M)\ (16.67)$$

M = milligrams of drug to be added to the base solution
D = dosage of drug in micrograms per kilogram per minute
W = body weight in kilograms
V = volume in milliliters of base solution
R = fluid rate in milliliters per hour
16.67 = conversion factor

Nursing consideration
It is important to make sure that the fluid used to dilute the drug is compatible with the medication. It is also important to make sure that if multiple medications are

administered via the same IV line all drugs are compatible. The Kings Guide to Parenteral Admixtures (www.kingguide.com) and the *Handbook of Injectable Drugs* by Trissel[15] are excellent resources for determining drug compatibility. Personnel administering the drugs should also have knowledge of potential side effects or adverse reactions.

RECUMBENT PATIENT CARE

Patients suffering from altered level of consciousness or neurologic, orthopedic, or traumatic problems can be recumbent for prolonged periods. Care of the recumbent patient can be challenging. Primary nursing goals are to minimize or prevent decubital ulcers (pressure sores), lung atelectasis, and aspiration pneumonia. In addition, supportive care must be addressed for bladder and bowel movement, skin care, and nutrition.

Decubital Ulcers

Decubital ulcers develop over bony prominences (points of the elbows, greater trochanter, and ischial tuberosities) as a result of continuous pressure and damage to the skin when the skin is compressed between a bone and an external surface (cage floor). Other factors that have been reported in the human literature to contribute to decubital ulcer formation include inadequate nutrition, moist skin, decreased sensory perception, and friction or shearing forces. Only the bottoms of the feet are made to withstand the continuous pressure of the body's weight. Patients in lateral recumbency for extended periods are at risk for the development of decubital ulcers. High-intensity pressure over a short period can create tissue damage just as low-intensity pressure over a long period can result in damage. Adequate nutrition is important for maintaining skin integrity. Protein deficiency and dehydration are linked to skin breakdown, decreased skin integrity, and delayed wound healing. Moistness can contribute to skin breakdown by macerating the surrounding skin, causing superficial erosion of the epidermis. Sources of moisture include urine, feces, and wound drainage. Decreased sensory perception occurs in the patient with altered mentation or some other neurologic deficit that prevents it from being able to recognize the cues that it needs to change body position. Friction and shearing forces may occur if a patient is dragged or pulled across a floor leading to disruption of skin integrity.

Decubital ulcer prevention

To achieve the nursing goals in the prevention of decubital ulcer formation, veterinary technicians can provide pressure relief, ensure appropriate nutritional support, keep the patient clean and dry, and enhance or maintain circulation. Bedding is an important factor in the prevention of decubital ulcers. Fleece pads and blankets work well to aid in pressure relief. Air (**Fig. 7**) and water mattresses have also been advocated for use in the prevention of decubital ulcers. It is also helpful to place the patient on padded grates, to prevent the patient from lying in urine-soaked fleece pads. If a patient becomes urine soaked, it should be bathed immediately; this prevents urine scalding. Clipping the fur in the inguinal and perineal regions helps to minimize urine scalding and fecal staining and facilitates proper skin care. Applying a waterproof barrier cream on clean dry skin aids in its protection. Disposable diapers (nappies) are excellent for absorbing urine and keeping the patient dry. Recumbent patients should be turned every 2 to 4 hours if they are not sternal. If sternal, the hips should be shifted to the opposite side. Pulling or dragging the patient across the floor should be avoided; rather the patient should be lifted and turned. If exercise is not contraindicated, range of motion (ROM) exercises and massage should be instituted. ROM

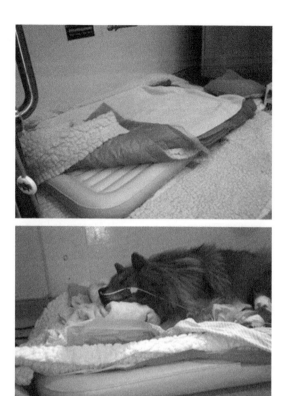

Fig. 7. Bedding for a recumbent patient; note the air mattress covered with fleece pads and absorbent covers.

exercises are indicated in nonambulatory or paretic patients. ROM exercises promote circulation and maintain flexibility and integrity of joints, muscles, and tendons. ROM exercises also affect articular cartilage, ligaments, fascia, blood vessels, and nerves in addition to joints, muscles, and tendons. ROM exercises are contraindicated in cases in which the patient has excessive pain or has undergone recent surgical repair. ROM exercises entail the movement of a joint or body segment through the maximum motion possible. Each joint or segment must be taken through its full ROM several times (10–20 repetitions) every 6 to 8 hours. The exercises can take the form of passive or active ROM. In the passive ROM form technique, the care giver provides the force needed to drive the motion. In the active form, the muscles of the patient are responsible for the motion. Massage is indicated to reduce stress and pain, muscle spasm, decreased ROM, recumbency, and contractures. If peripheral edema is present, massage may be helpful in reducing the edema. In addition to relieving stress, pain, and muscle spasm, it maintains tissue perfusion and sensory input to the spinal cord.

Lung Atelectasis

Atelectasis is the collapse of alveoli. As a result of the collapsed alveoli, there is a reduction in the size of the affected lung lobes. Although there are several causes for atelectasis, the main reason in the recumbent patient is compression of the alveoli. It is often caused by pressure on the chest wall and frequently occurs in large breed or obese dogs recumbent on one side for prolonged periods. The patient may display signs of increased respiratory rate, effort, and cough. It may also have dull lung sounds or crackles. Oxygen saturation and arterial oxygen levels may show variable degrees of hypoxemia.

Prevention and management of atelectasis

If there are any constricting bandages on the patient, they should be removed. The patient is turned or repositioned every 2 to 4 hours and ideally would be kept sternal and have the hips turned every 2 hours. If possible, the patient should be helped to stand or even take a short walk to encourage deeper breaths. Coupage also encourages deeper breaths. If the patient is hypoxemic, oxygen is administered.

Aspiration Pneumonia

Aspiration pneumonia is the result of inhalation of fluid that comes from the contents of the gastric or oral cavities. There are many risk factors for aspiration pneumonia, including heavy sedation or anesthesia, impaired protective airway reflexes (ie, impaired consciousness), or weakness, paresis, or paralysis. Recumbent patients that are being fed enterally are also predisposed to aspiration pneumonia.[16,17]

Prevention and management of aspiration pneumonia

Prevention can be a challenge; it is important to recognize those patients at risk for aspiration pneumonia and develop strategies to minimize the risk. If the patient has an impaired gag reflex, it must be intubated and a plan to initiate artificial airway management instituted. It is beneficial to avoid keeping the patient's head elevated unless contraindicated (ie, patients with head trauma); head elevation may put the patient at risk for reflux and aspiration. At-risk patients may benefit from prophylactic therapy to reduce the incidence of gastric reflux; however, reviews of this practice in both the human and veterinary literature are mixed.[18] Prokinetics, protein pump inhibitors, and histamine antagonist have all been used. Little morbidity has been associated with these drugs; the potential benefit associated with the administration may warrant consideration.

Oxygen therapy is indicated when aspiration pneumonia results in hypoxemia or respiratory distress. If the patient has an elevated $Paco_2$ approaching 60 mm Hg or greater or the patient is working so hard to breathe that it exhausts itself, mechanical ventilation is indicated. Antimicrobials are used in the treatment of aspiration pneumonia, and the selection is based on culture and susceptibility testing of either transtracheal wash or bronchial alveolar lavage. In the absence of culture results, empirical dosing with broad-spectrum antimicrobials is indicated. Local resistance profiles should be taken into consideration with empirical dosing. Nebulization and coupage are commonly used in veterinary medicine, the goal being to humidify secretions and promote removal. In addition to nebulization and coupage, other supportive therapies include bronchodilators and glucocorticoids. Despite the supportive therapies not showing any correlation with survival, the importance of supportive care in patients with aspiration pneumonia should not be underestimated.[19]

Bladder and Bowel Maintenance

Ideally, the patient urinates voluntarily. Taking the canine patient outside can help stimulate and promote urination. Many patients are reluctant to urinate lying down; if the patient has difficulty standing, supporting the patient while encouraging urination is beneficial. If the patient does not urinate voluntarily, attempts need to be made to manually express the bladder. Bladder expression should be performed 3 to 4 times a day. Once the bladder is palpated, steady pressure is applied; several seconds may be required to overcome the sphincter tone. Sudden movements may cause the patient to tense its abdomen. Two hands may be used in the large breed patient and 1 hand in cats and small breed dogs. If manual expression is difficult or painful, then an aseptically placed indwelling or intermittent urinary catheter may be used. There are pros and cons for each technique. One study of dogs with intervertebral disc disease stated that treatment for urinary bladder management should be limited where possible and no method of treatment is preferred.[20] Documentation should be made regarding bladder size, the act of urination, and the amount, color, and odor of urine.

Animals reflexively defecate when the rectal area is stimulated (internally or externally). In some instances, it may be necessary to administer an enema or digitally remove the feces. If the animal has loose stool or diarrhea, the insertion in the rectum of a Foley catheter that is attached to a closed urinary collection system helps to keep the patient clean. In addition, the diarrhea can be quantitated. Changing the diet to a low-residue diet can decrease stool volume; that coupled with establishing a routine can be helpful in controlling the frequency of defecation.

Nutrition

Nutrition is an important factor that must be addressed in all patients (see Peri-Surgical Nutrition: Perspectives and Perceptions by Frye and colleagues elsewhere in this issue). The American Animal Hospital Association has developed nutritional assessment guidelines[21] that aid in the development of a nutrition plan for the ill patient. The benefits of nutritional support are well known; in the recumbent patient nutrition plays a vital role in maintaining skin integrity.

Food and water should be placed within easy reach of the patient. The patient should be fed its daily caloric requirements. Recumbent patients may not be willing to eat on their own and may require hand feeding. Patients should be maintained in sternal recumbency for feeding and for at least 15 minutes after feeding. If the patient is unable to take food orally, then enteral or parental feeding must be considered. Patients with feeding tubes may be at increased risk of aspiration due to gastric distension and atony following feeding.

RENAL NURSING CARE
Ins and Outs

For the purposes of this discussion, the focus in renal nursing is primarily on fluid balance (see Assessment of Fluid Balance and the Approach to Fluid Therapy in the Perioperative Patient by Boller and Boller elsewhere in this issue). Ins and outs should be monitored at regular intervals over the course of 24 hours. The patient's condition dictates the frequency at which fluid balance is assessed. Ins (IV fluids, IV medications, water, and liquid feedings) and outs (urine, diarrhea, vomitus, gastric suctioning, and fluid from body cavities) can be monitored as frequently as every hour to as infrequently as every 8 hours. Ideally, the ins should equal the outs. If the input exceeds the output, the patient is at risk for fluid overload; if the output exceeds the input, the patient is at risk for dehydration. Body weight is an excellent way to assess fluid balance, as acute changes in body weight are usually due to fluid gains or fluid losses. For example, if a patient weighed 15 kg at the start of fluid therapy and weighs 15.3 kg 6 hours later, it has gained 300 mL of fluid.

Quantifying Urine Production

Normal urine output is 1 to 2 mL/kg/h. A patient with a urine production of less than 0.25 mL/kg/h and less than 0.08 mL/kg/h is considered oliguric and anuric, respectively. Placement of an indwelling urinary catheter along with a closed urinary collection system is the most accurate way to quantify urine production. However, indwelling urinary catheters place the patient at risk for developing a urinary tract infection (UTI). The benefits versus the risks of the indwelling urinary catheter must be considered. If the patient is nonambulatory, a diaper (nappies) can be placed underneath the patient to catch the urine. In some cases, a diaper can actually be placed on the patient to wear (**Fig. 8**). The diaper should be weighed before placing it underneath or on the patient. The difference between the wet weight and dry weight (in grams) equals the volume in milliliters of urine produced.

Urinary Catheter Care and Maintenance

Urinary catheter care
The primary goal of urinary catheter care is to minimize the risk of development of a UTI. It has been suggested that placement of an indwelling urinary catheter in dogs is associated with a low risk of catheter-associated UTI during the first 3 days after catheter placement, provided that adequate precautions are taken for aseptic catheter placement and maintenance.[22] Urinary catheter care is performed every 8 hours or as needed. It entails cleaning the prepuce or vulva and its surrounding area with a mild soap followed by a water rinse. The vulvar or preputial area is then flushed with 2 to 10 mL (depending on patient size) of 0.05% chlorhexidine solution (6 mL chlorhexidine in 250 mL sterile water). The urinary catheter itself should be kept clean, especially in the female patient where the vulva is in close proximity to the rectum.

Urinary collection system
The urinary catheter should be attached to a collection system. By maintaining a closed collection system the chance of a UTI is decreased. The urinary catheter should not be disconnected from the collection system and should be drained only every 4 to 6 hours rather than hourly. Urinary collection bags may be obtained commercially (closed system), or empty sterile IV bags (open system) can be used. One study showed that used IV bags that were properly stored (<7 days, had not contained dextrose, stoppered with an administration set spike or 1-mL syringe and stored in a cabinet) were not a source of aerobic bacterial contamination when used as a part of a urinary collection system.[23] The type of urinary collection system

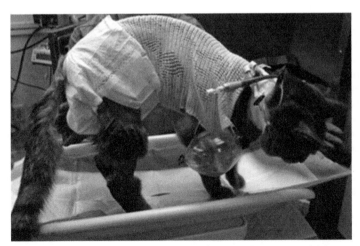

Fig. 8. Placement of a diaper on a patient to catch urine; this is also useful for quantitating urine.

(closed vs open) was not associated with the likelihood of developing nosocomial bacteriuria in a recent study.[24]

Changing indwelling catheters or drainage bags at routine, fixed intervals is not recommended. Rather, it is suggested to change catheters and drainage bags based on clinical indications such as infection and obstruction or when the closed system is compromised.[25]

SUMMARY

The veterinary technician must have an understanding and working knowledge of a variety of nursing care techniques. The technician should know what it takes to perform the technique, be aware of risk factors and potential complications, and know what action is to be taken if the complication is encountered. As a part of nursing care, technicians should constantly evaluate the patient's condition and ask if the nursing goals are being met and if risk factors are turning into complications. It is better to be proactive rather than reactive to potential complications. "If you don't look, you won't see."

REFERENCES

1. Rockett J, Lattanzio C, Anderson K. Veterinary technician practice model and documentation. In: Rockett J, Lattanzio C, Anderson K, editors. Patient assessment, intervention and documentation for the veterinary technician. New York: Delmar Cengage Learning; 2009. p. 1–34.
2. Rockett J, Lattanzio C, Anderson K. Technician evaluations with suggested interventions. In: Rockett J, Lattanzio C, Anderson K, editors. Patient assessment, intervention and documentation for the veterinary technician. New York: Delmar Cengage Learning; 2009. p. 53–121.
3. Nance-Floyd B. Tracheostomy care: an evidence-based guide to suctioning and dressing changes. Am Nurse Today 2011;6(7):14–6.
4. Fossum TW. Surgery of the lower respiratory system: pleural cavity and diaphragm. In: Fossum TW, Dewey CW, Horn CV, et al, editors. Small animal surgery. 4th edition. St Louis (MO): Elsevier; 2013. p. 991–1032.
5. Monnet E. Pyothorax. In: King LG, editor. Textbook of respiratory disease in dogs and cat. St Louis (MO): Saunders; 2004. p. 605–10.
6. Gordon PA, Norton JM, Guerra JM, et al. Positioning of chest tubes: effects on pressure and drainage. Am J Crit Care 1997;6(1):33–8.
7. Schmelz JO, Johnson D, Norton JM, et al. Effects of position of chest drainage tube on volume drained and pressure. Am J Crit Care 1999;8(5):319–23.
8. American College of Veterinary Anesthesiologist. Recommendations for monitoring anesthetized veterinary patients. J Am Vet Med Assoc 1995;206(7):936–7.
9. American College of Veterinary Anesthesiologist Analgesia Web site ACVA Monitoring Guidelines Update, 2009 Recommendations for monitoring the anesthetized veterinary patient. Available at: www.acvaa.org/Index. Accessed February 14, 2015.
10. Center for Disease Control Web site. Guidelines for the prevention of intravascular related infections. Available at: www.cdc.gov/hicpac/pdf/guidelines/bsi-guidelines-2011.pdf. Accessed March 12, 2015.
11. Mathews KA, Brooks MJ, Valliant AE. A prospective study of intravenous catheter contamination. J Vet Emerg Crit Care (San Antonio) 1996;6:33.
12. Arnts IJ, Heijnen JA, Wilbers HT, et al. Effectiveness of heparin solution versus normal saline in maintaining patency of intravenous in neonates: a double blind randomized controlled study. J Adv Nurs 2011;67(12):2677–85.

13. Wang R, Luo O, He L, et al. Preservative free 0.9% sodium chloride for flushing and locking peripheral intravenous devices: a prospective control trial. J Evid Based Med 2012;5(4):205–8.

14. Ueda Y, Odunayo A, Mann FA. Comparison of heparinized saline and 0.9% sodium chloride for maintaining peripheral intravenous catheter patency in dogs. J Vet Emerg Crit Care (San Antonio) 2013;23(5):517–22.

15. Trissel LA. Handbook of injectable drugs. 16th edition. Bethesda (MD): American Society of Health-System Pharmacists; 2010.

16. Marik PE, Zaloga GP. Gastric versus post-pyloric feeding: a systematic review. Crit Care 2002;7(3):R46–51.

17. Kazi N, Mobarhan S. Enteral feeding associated gastroesophageal reflux and aspiration pneumonia: a review. Nutr Rev 1996;54:324–8.

18. Schulze HM, Rahilly LJ. Aspiration pneumonia in dogs: pathophysiology, prevention, and diagnosis. Compend Contin Educ Vet 2012;34:E5.

19. Tart KM, Babski DM, Lee JA. Potential risk, prognostic indicators, and diagnostic and treatment modalities affecting survival in dogs with presumptive aspiration pneumonia: 125 cases (2005-2008). J Vet Emerg Crit Care (San Antonio) 2010; 20(3):319–29.

20. Bubenik L, Hosgood G. Urinary tract infection in dogs with thoracolumbar intervertebral disc herniation and urinary bladder dysfunction managed by manual expression, indwelling catheterization or intermittent catheterization. Vet Surg 2008;37:791–800.

21. Baldwin K, Bartges L, Buffington T, et al. AAHA nutritional guidelines for the dog and cat. J Am Anim Hosp Assoc 2010;46:285–96.

22. Smarick SD, Haskins SC, Aldrich J, et al. Incidence of catheter-associated urinary tract infection among dogs in a small animal intensive care unit. J Am Vet Med Assoc 2004;224(12):1936–40.

23. Barrett M, Campbell VL. Aerobic bacterial culture of used intravenous fluid bags intended for use as urine collection reservoirs. J Am Anim Hosp Assoc 2008;44:2–4.

24. Sullivan LA, Campbell VL, Onuma SC. Evaluation of open versus closed urine collection systems and development of nosocomial bacteriuria in dogs. J Am Vet Med Assoc 2010;237(2):187–90.

25. Center for Disease Control. Guidelines for the prevention of catheter-associated urinary tract infection, 2009. 2009. Available at: www.cdc.gov/hicpac/cauti/001_cauti.html. Accessed March 12, 2015.

Wound Care

Ingrid M. Balsa, DVM, William T.N. Culp, VMD*

KEYWORDS

• Wound management • Wound healing • Bandage • Dressing

KEY POINTS

• Wound healing generally progresses through inflammatory, repair, and maturation phases.
• If wound healing is not progressing as expected, the wound management technique should be reassessed and the patient evaluated for causes of delays in wound healing.
• Delays in wound healing may be caused by infection, wound location, poor nutritional status of the patient, certain medications, and underlying metabolic diseases.
• The nature of the wound should dictate whether closure is attempted immediately, later, or never, allowing the wound to heal by second intention.
• The management of a wound and the bandage used for the wound must evolve over time as the wound progresses through stages of healing.

INTRODUCTION

Wound care in veterinary medicine has changed significantly over the past 25 years owing to an enhanced understanding of the cellular processes of wound healing. Appropriate patient wound care must take into account the normal process of wound healing, as well as patient factors and comorbidities. One must also understand the myriad of wound care products available, the phase of wound healing in which they are most likely to be helpful, and in which phases they may delay or interfere with healing. All wounds, from surgical incisions to puncture wounds to traumatic degloving injuries, undergo the same healing process. Therefore, wound care that does not take patient factors into account and provide appropriate wound therapy may delay the process of successful wound healing and the return of normal structure and function of the skin.[1]

PHASES OF WOUND HEALING

Although phases of wound healing are delineated as separate entities for ease of discussion, phases may overlap and a wound may have areas that are in different

The authors have nothing to disclose.
Department of Surgical and Radiological Sciences, University of California, Davis, One Shields Drive, Davis, CA 95616, USA
* Corresponding author.
E-mail address: wculp@ucdavis.edu

phases at any given time. The phases of wound healing begin immediately after development of the wound or incision and the timeline given below represents a standard, noninfected skin wound in an otherwise healthy patient.

Inflammatory Phase: Time 0

At the time of wounding, vasoconstriction occurs initially owing to endothelin production and the release of epinephrine, norepinephrine and prostaglandins.[2] However, within 5 to 10 minutes there is an increase in vascular permeability that brings about the classic signs of inflammation: redness, edema, heat, and pain. This increased vascular permeability facilitates chemotaxis of circulatory cells and release of cytokines and growth factors from activated platelets. Bleeding is considered a protective mechanism because it cleans the wound and fills the defect. The injured cells release thromboplastin, which initiates the extrinsic pathway of the coagulation cascade.

Platelet aggregation and coagulation along with cross-linking of fibrin and fibronectin leads to clot formation and formation of a scaffold.[3] Platelets release chemoattractants and growth factors that are important in recruiting other important cells to allow for the progression of wound healing (**Table 1**). When subdivided into a debridement phase, the inflammatory phase is considered complete when white blood cells leaking from blood vessels enter the wound.

Debridement Phase: Time 6 to 12 Hours After Wound Initiation

The debridement phase is often considered part of the inflammatory phase, but is characterized by the migration of white blood cells, specifically neutrophils and monocytes, into the wound. Neutrophils phagocytize organisms and debris contaminating the wound. Degenerating neutrophils release enzymes and free radicals that kill bacteria and break down extracellular and necrotic debris.

Monocytes, which transform into macrophages in response to the extracellular matrix, are essential for wound healing because they are responsible for synthesizing and secreting the growth factors responsible for tissue formation and remodeling. Macrophages phagocytize other phagocytes as well as bacteria and damaged tissue. Macrophages also stimulate angiogenesis, recruit mesenchymal cells, and modulate matrix production in wounds. In the absence of macrophages, wound healing and the tensile strength of the wound are impaired (**Fig. 1A1, B1**).

Table 1 Growth factor important in wound healing	
Growth Factor	**Origin**
Platelet-derived growth factor (PDGF)	Platelets, macrophages, endothelial cells, keratinocytes
Transforming growth factor-α (TGF-α)	Macrophages, T-lymphocytes, keratinocytes
Transforming growth factor-β (TGF-β)	Platelets, T-lymphocytes, macrophages, endothelial cells, keratinocytes, fibroblasts
Epidermal growth factor (EGF)	Platelets, macrophages
Vascular endothelial growth factor (VEGF)	Keratinocytes
Fibroblast growth factor (FGF)	Macrophages, mast cells, T-lymphocytes, endothelial cells and fibroblasts

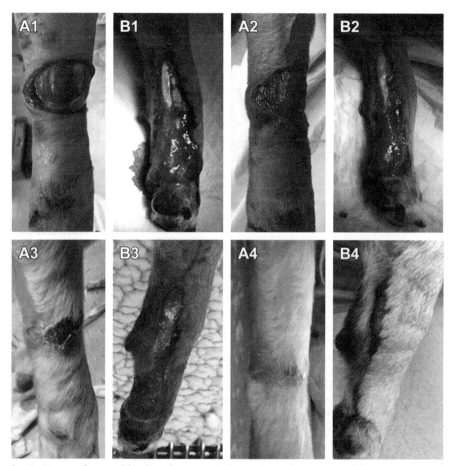

Fig. 1. Stages of wound healing for a surgical resection of a sarcoma (A) versus traumatic wound (B) by second intention healing. (A1, B1) Inflammatory phase, day 1. (A2, B2) Repair phase, at days 12 and 4, respectively. (A3, B3) Late repair phase, days 34 and 7, respectively. (A4, B4) Maturation phase, days 41 and 120, respectively.

Repair Phase (Proliferation Phase): 3 to 12 Days After Wound Initiation

This phase is composed of 3 distinct processes, namely, fibroplasia, angiogenesis, and epithelialization (see **Fig. 1**A2, B2). The prominent cell types are fibroblasts, endothelial cells, and epithelial cells.[4]

Fibroplasia

Fibroblasts originate from undifferentiated mesenchymal cells present in connective tissue surrounding the wound; they migrate along fibrin strands in the fibrin clot. Fibroblast proliferation is stimulated primarily by macrophages, cytokines and extracellular matrix molecules such as platelet-derived growth factor, transforming growth factor (TGF)-β and endothelial growth factor. Fibroblast cell binding and movement are stimulated by TGF-β and the subsequent production of fibronectin. The wound environment, slight acidity, and tissue oxygen content also stimulates fibroblast proliferation and therefore collagen synthesis.

The fibroblasts create elastin, collagen, and proteoglycans that are arranged initially in a haphazard pattern. At approximately day 5 of healing, tension on the wound forces fibroblasts, fibers, and capillaries to orient parallel to the wound edges. Fibrin is remodeled and increased collagen appears in the wounds. As collagen content increases in the wound, the number of fibroblasts decrease as does the rate of collagen synthesis. Maximum collagen content is reached at approximately 2 to 3 weeks after the initiation of wound healing.

Angiogenesis

Capillaries enter the wound just behind the fibroblasts and grow from existing vasculature. Angiogenesis is stimulated by cytokines, specifically basic fibroblast growth factor, vascular endothelial cell growth factor, endothelial growth factor, and TGF-β, among others. The new capillaries, fibroblasts, fibrous tissue, and an active extracellular matrix form the granulation tissue which is normally present no sooner than 4 days after wounding.[5] The formation of granulation tissue is a benchmark in wound healing because it is resistant to infection, plays a role in wound contraction, and provides a scaffold for epithelialization (see **Fig. 1**A3, B3).

Epithelialization

In the case of full-thickness wounds, the basement membrane of the epidermis is not left intact. Therefore, epithelialization must occur from the wound edges. Epithelial cells proliferate at the wound edge in response to cytokines, endothelial growth factor, and TGF-α, secreted by platelets and macrophages. Basal epithelial cells migrate out from the edge of the wound. This migration may take weeks depending on the size of the wound, and initially, the coverage is thin and fragile. Migration ends when epithelial cells come into contact with each other (contact inhibition). Proliferation and differentiation of cells then takes place to form a new basement membrane; this does not include the formation of new adnexa and therefore initially, and in some cases permanently, the skin remains hairless. The repair phase is generally considered complete when the epidermis is reestablished across the granulation bed.

Maturation Phase (Remodeling Phase): 7 Days to Several Months after Wound Initiation

The main event during this phase is the strengthening of the newly formed collagen. Over time, collagen fibers become thicker and progressively more cross-linked. They align with the tension lines of the body and nonfunctionally oriented fibers are degraded. Remaining fibroblasts in the wound differentiate into myofibroblasts under the influence of TGF-β. Myofibroblasts are contractile and therefore can continue to pull the wound edges together. The greatest increase in wound strength occurs in the first 7 days of this phase or approximately 1 to 2 weeks from the time of wounding, because this is the time of greatest collagen deposition.[6] The maturation phase may continue for months, eventually leaving a scar that is 80% of the tissue's original strength before wounding (see **Fig. 1**A4, B4).[4,6,7]

FACTORS AFFECTING WOUND HEALING
Infection

Care should be taken to differentiate between a wound infection and wound contamination. Contamination is the presence of microorganisms in the wound without a host response; contamination can also include gross debris. Infection is the presence of microorganisms at or above the level of 10^5 per gram of tissue.[4]

Surgical site infections (SSI) are defined as any infection that develops in the operative site after an operative procedure.[8] SSI include both incisional and organ/cavity infections. Incisional infections are subdivided into superficial, which involve the skin and subcutis, or deep, which involve the underlying musculature. Infections that occur in areas other than the body wall are classified as organ/space infection.[9] A recent retrospective paper reported an overall incidence of 3% for SSI in a veterinary hospital. Of those, 42% were superficial, 50% were deep, and 8% were organ/space. The most commonly cultured organism was *Staphylococci* (74%).[10]

Prevention of SSI relies on appropriate preparation of the patient skin with regard to clipping and scrubbing as well as surgical team preparation. In humans, there is significant evidence that hair removal of any kind increases the chance of an SSI. In veterinary medicine, hair removal is necessary owing to the amount of hair our patients have, and should be done with clippers immediately before surgery; razors should not be used routinely.[11–13] When hair is clipped around wounds, the wound should either be closed temporarily or protected from contamination by applying a sterile, water-soluble lubricant. Maintaining normothermia, normal blood pressure, normoglycemia, and appropriate tissue oxygenation have all been recommended as a means of reducing the risk of SSI.[10,12]

Location

Motion and tension are limits to wound healing that are inherent in certain locations on the body, but may play a role anywhere in the body with a large enough defect. Motion can lead to increased tension when a joint is moved through its normal range of motion. If needed, a bandage can minimize motion. Tension can lead to wound dehiscence/suture pull-out and ischemia and necrosis of the surrounding skin.[14] Excessive tension when closing wounds on the distal limbs can lead to compression of blood and lymphatic vessels, causing congestion and swelling of the limb, requiring the wound to be reopened, and wound healing by second intention.

Wounds in the perianal, oral, or other locations with an increased bacterial burden are often managed as open wounds because closure is more likely to result in infection and failure from dehiscence.

Nutrition

Nutrition must be taken into account in postoperative patients, because the healing of large wounds places the animal in a catabolic state. Malnourished animals or animals that have comorbidities that cause their serum protein to be less than 2.0 g/dL may have decreased wound healing and strength.[15] Diets deficient in protein have been demonstrated to delay wound healing.[16] Care should be taken to ensure proper caloric and protein intake in animals with large or chronic wounds.

Medications

Many medications may play a role in wound healing. Steroids and chemotherapeutic agents are the 2 medications that typically receive the most attention. Steroids have been shown to cause epidermal and granulation tissue atrophy, delay wound healing, and reduce wound tensile strength.[17,18] Chemotherapeutic agents may result in delays in wound healing owing to their mechanism of action; they attack rapidly dividing cells and have been shown to affect fibroblast proliferation and wound strength.[19,20] Nonsteroidal anti-inflammatory medications have also been investigated with regard to their effects on wound healing, because inflammation is the first step in normal wound healing. These medications have not been found to alter the rate of wound healing significantly.[17,21,22]

Metabolic Diseases

Hyperadrenocorticism, diabetes mellitus, and uremia have all been show to delay wound healing. In human medicine and in animal models, diabetes mellitus has been shown to decrease the inflammatory response, impair chemotaxis, and decrease bacterial killing.[4] However, no reports in veterinary medicine have connected diabetes mellitus with decreased wound healing in clinical patients. In 1 veterinary retrospective study, patients with an endocrinopathy had a significant increase in the risk of development of an SSI.[23]

Radiation Therapy

Radiation therapy affects tissue, fibroblasts, and growth factor production, as well as local vasculature. The decrease in vasculature at a site owing to fibrotic microangiopathy may decrease oxygen content to a level below what is needed for normal wound healing. In 1 study, 70% of dogs that underwent radiation therapy and a flap procedure for reconstruction after tumor resection had at least 2 complications, with dehiscence being the most common complication. However, use of flaps was considered successful in 85% of the patients.[24]

Species Differences

Dogs and cats have differences in wound healing that may be in part to differences in cutaneous angiosomes. Dogs have a greater density of collateral subcutaneous trunk vessels, which increases tissue perfusion.[25]

With regard to primary wound healing, cat wounds are only half as strong as dog wounds at day 7. During the first week, cats also have decreased cutaneous perfusion compared with dogs; however, by week 2 there does not seem to be a perfusion difference.[26] For these reasons, some authors suggest that skin sutures in cats be left in place longer than the traditional 10 to 14 days.[4] With regard to second intention healing, cats produce less granulation tissue than dogs and this tissue is located peripherally in the wound as compared with the centrally located granulation tissue of dogs. This may result in cats being slower to heal and slower to contract; therefore, judicious debridement of subcutaneous fat should be performed to avoid devitalization of skin.[25,27]

WOUND CARE
Lavage

Lavage of wounds to rid the wound of contamination is an important first step and many times allows for further evaluation of the wound. The functions of lavage have been stated as removal of devitalized tissue, reduction of bacterial contamination, and removal of gross debris.[28] Multiple lavage solutions have been suggested with or without the addition of antiseptics, such as povidone iodine. The addition of antiseptics has not been found to enhance the benefits of lavage.[29] Ultimately, lavage of a high volume of fluid delivered via a large syringe and 18-gauge catheter has been recommended.[30] However, other studies have shown that the ideal wound lavage pressure is best reached with a 1 L bag pressurized to 300 mm Hg and the gauge of needle was not an important factor for altering lavage pressure.[31] The exact volume to be delivered has not been elucidated although an estimate of 50 to 100 mL per cm of laceration or square centimeter of wound has been suggested.[29]

With regard to the ideal solution, phosphate-buffered saline or lactated Ringer's solution should be used to lavage the wound until it is free of gross debris if possible. Use of sterile tap water and prolonged exposure to normal saline have both been found to be cytotoxic to fibroblasts in vitro and therefore cannot be recommend as a first choice lavage solution.[32] Alternatively, if no other solution is available, lavage of wounds with tap water has not been shown to increase the incidence of infection and may decrease it based on a systematic review of the human literature.[33]

Debridement

The purpose of debridement is to remove necrotic or damaged tissue that may delay healing and to ensure that the wound bed and edges have appropriate blood flow. This can be done surgically, via bandage debridement, with biosurgical debridement or with the addition of enzymatic agents for debridement.

Surgical debridement can either be selective (layered), in which devitalized tissue is removed, sparing tendons, nerves, and large blood vessels or may be performed en bloc, in which the entire wound is removed as a single piece of tissue. With selective surgical debridement, fat should be resected liberally for the reasons described; however, care must be taken not to damage the subdermal plexus and the vascular supply to the skin. Surgical debridement is appropriate for both primary and delayed closures as well as healing by second intention.

Bandage debridement with wet-to-dry or dry-to-dry bandages has fallen out of favor owing to the nonselective debridement that occurs when the contact layer is removed. This is especially of concern during the proliferative phase when granulation tissue can be debrided, delaying healing. Bandage debridement should only be used during the inflammatory phase of wound healing, if ever, and in wounds being managed with a delayed closure or healing by second intention.

Biosurgical debridement uses green bottle fly larvae (Lucilia sericata), which are sterile and specially bred medical maggots. Maggot therapy is best used in necrotic, moist, chronic wounds. The benefits include removal of necrotic tissue, disinfection of wound, and promotion of granulation tissue formation. Current recommendations are for 5 to 10 maggots per cm^2 of wound; the maggots should be left undisturbed for 1 to 3 days before bandage change.[34]

Finally, autolytic debridement is not a purposeful debridement on the part of the veterinarian, but rather is the natural process that will take place in a moist wound environment in which the enzymes present in the wound fluid debride necrotic tissue.

Antibiotic Coverage

Ideally, a culture sample appropriate to the wound type is taken at the time of wounding but after the area is lavaged. A swab of the wound bed may culture contaminants and therefore a tissue culture is preferred. Although in most cases empiric antibiotic therapy is started before culture results, once the results are known the culture will guide antibiotic therapy in the future, particularly if there is a delay in healing or evidence of infection.

The use of perioperative antibiotics should be directed at the expected pathogens and administered between 0 and 60 minutes before making an incision to maximize blood levels.[12,35] These antibiotics should be redosed depending on the length of the procedure and the amount of blood loss; more blood loss requires more frequent redosing.[12]

Generally, topical antibiotic therapy can be used to prevent bacterial colonization and systemic antibiotics should be reserved for cases of infection (**Table 2**). Topical antibiotics tend to be broad spectrum and are therefore appropriate for contaminated, traumatic wounds. Topical agents with antimicrobial properties include ointments, silver-based dressings, and hyperosmotic dressings (hypertonic saline, dextran soaked, sugar, honey).

Table 2	
Wound classification system	
Class	**Description**
Class I: Clean	Surgical wound in which no inflammation is encountered and the respiratory, alimentary, genital, or urinary tracts are not entered. Most often closed primarily with or without appropriate drainage.
Class II: Clean–contaminated	Surgical wound in which the respiratory, alimentary, genital, or urinary tracts are entered without unusual contamination or evidence of infection or break in sterile technique.
Class III: Contaminated	Open, fresh, accidental wounds. Surgical wound with major breaks in sterile techniques. Gross spillage from gastrointestinal tract. Incisions with acute, nonpurulent inflammation.
Class IV: Dirty–infected	Old traumatic wounds with retained devitalized tissue and/or existing infection or perforated viscera.

Modified from Garner JS. CDC guideline for prevention of surgical wound infections, 1985. Supersedes guideline for prevention of surgical wound infections published in 1982 (Originally published in 1995). Revised. Infect Control 1986;7(3):193–200; and Simmons BP. Guideline for prevention of surgical wound infections. Infect Control 1982;3:185–96.

Antibiotic ointments are most commonly a combination of bacitracin zinc, neomycin sulfate, and polymixin B sulfate. These ointments tend to be well-tolerated and have the added benefit of keeping the wound bed moist.

Silver-based dressings arose from the use of silver sulfadiazine (1%) ointment as a topical antibacterial agent. Silver is a broad-spectrum antibiotic that has effects against many bacteria including *Pseudomonas* as well as certain fungal pathogens. Silver sulfadiazine has now largely been replaced by slow-release silver-impregnated dressings, which are available in a variety of formulas.[36] Silver dressings may result in a surface exudate that is similar in appearance to infection with *Pseudomonas*; lavage of the wound bed is required to determine the true character of the granulation tissue.

Hyperosmotic dressings function by dehydrating and killing microorganisms. Care must be taken to place these dressings only in the wound bed, because this same dehydration can occur to healthy skin surrounding the wound causing detrimental effects.

The antimicrobial properties of honey likely stem from the enzymatic production of low levels of hydrogen peroxide; alternatively it may also be owing to the very low pH of honey or the high osmolality (similar to sugar dressings).[37] Additionally, medical grade honey is rated by its inhibin effect, which seems to encompass antimicrobial properties other than the production of hydrogen peroxide that have not yet been elucidated fully. Honey has also been advocated in wound management because it creates a moist wound environment, thereby increasing autolytic debridement and enhancing granulation tissue formation and epithelialization. The high viscosity of honey provides a protective barrier from the environment.

Wound Environment

Regardless of the type of closure that is appropriate for an individual wound, there is increasing interest in maintaining a moist wound environment. Although rarely done in clinical patients, some authors suggest maintaining a moist environment even in primary closure cases with the application of a triple antibiotic ointment over the incision.[4] More commonly, the desire to maintain a moist environment occurs with open wound management. A moist environment is thought to limit the opportunity for infection, because more neutrophils are present in moist wounds because these are not trapped in scabs, and epithelialization occurs more rapidly because epithelial cells do not need to migrate beneath a scab. Additionally, wound fluid is thought to facilitate autolytic debridement of necrotic tissue owing to endogenous enzymes. Wound fluid also contains cytokines and growth factors that stimulate fibroplasia and epithelialization, depending on the phase of wound healing. Wound fluid may also contain antibiotics if the animal is receiving systemic antibiotics.

WOUND CLOSURE

Before attempting a primary or delayed closure, assessment of the skin's viability must be made. This is done clinically by assessing skin color, evidence of bleeding, and the presence of pain sensation and warmth. Nonviable skin is often less supple and has more of a leathery feeling than viable skin. Nonviable skin will not have capillary bleeding at the wound edges and is blue, black, or white in appearance. Skin may 'declare' itself viable or nonviable over the course of several days depending on the extent and type of injury sustained.

Primary Closure

Primary closure of a wound is most appropriate for wounds that are classified as freshly incised, clean, or clean-contaminated. If a traumatic wound is treated within 6 hours of injury and the wound edges seem to be vascularized, it is also reasonable to attempt a primary closure. This time frame is limited by the multiplication of bacteria, because ideally the wound would be closed before the bacterial population exceeds 10^5 organisms per gram of tissue, after which time the chance for infection increases.[4]

Closure techniques and suture type may depend on the depth of the wound and patient comorbidities, as described. If there is reason to believe wound healing may be delayed, use of a slowly absorbable suture and interrupted pattern may be beneficial for holding strength.

Management of these wounds after closure is usually minimal; epithelialization should proceed across the minimal epidermal gap. Incisions should be kept clean. Analgesia is often the main concern and can be achieved with nonsteroidal antiinflammatory medications, local anesthetic agents, and cold compresses. Systemic opioids may be needed for larger wounds or surgeries.

Delayed Primary or Secondary Closure

Delayed primary closure is primary closure of a wound 3 to 5 days after wounding, whereas secondary closure is closure of the wound beyond that time point. Generally, more contaminated wounds and those with more trauma to the surrounding tissue require longer open wound management. Ultimately, secondary closure is performed over a bed of granulation tissue.[4] These methods should be considered for all crushing injuries, as the declaration of skin may continue for 3 to 7 days after insult, and for all previously dehisced incisions, because there is an increased bacterial burden, among many other wound types.

Second Intention Healing

Second intention healing occurs when a wound is allowed to progress through the stages of wound healing and epithelialization without operative intervention. All wounds can be managed this way; however, this may be impractical with very large wounds or in patients with multiple comorbidities (see **Fig. 1**).

Negative Pressure Wound Therapy

Negative pressure wound therapy (NPWT) has been suggested to increase the formation of granulation tissue, reduce bacterial load, increase blood flow, decrease hematoma and seroma formation, and increase cytokines and growth factors.[38,39] Some of these factors have been investigated in randomized, blinded, prospective studies and others are based more on clinical observation than scientific data. NPTW was originally investigated in veterinary medicine for use over traumatic wounds; however, studies have shown use with grafts and flaps as well as in cases of primary closure.[40,41]

NPWT can be used as a temporary measure in wounds that go on to heal by second intention or for wounds in which delayed primary closure is the ultimate goal.[42] The wound is treated initially with lavage and debridement of necrotic tissue. The NPWT system is then placed and maintained at a pressure of approximately −125 mm Hg. Ideally, NPWT is used in the inflammatory and early repair phases. Once granulation tissue is present, NPWT may delay wound epithelialization and contraction.[38]

Management benefits of NPWT include less frequent bandage changes than traditional bandages. When used in less tolerant animals, general anesthesia may be required for NPWT bandage changes, but at a minimum, sedation is necessary for most animals. The cost of an NPWT system and the cost of the materials should be taken into account when planning wound management.

DRAINS

The placement of a drain should be considered when a contaminated or dirty–infected wound is closed to allow for the continuation of drainage of blood and serum, which could otherwise be trapped and allow for bacterial proliferation. Additionally, the placement of a drain could be considered whenever there is an unusually large amount of dead space regardless of the classification of the wound. Drains should not lie directly under the wound closure or incision, nor exit from the wound itself. Most drains can be removed in 3 to 5 days when fluid accumulation has decreased and reached a steady state. A complication of drain placement includes nosocomial infections and, therefore, the exit sites of the drains should be kept covered if possible.[43]

Drains may be classified as either passive (eg, Penrose drain) or active (eg, Jackson–Pratt drain). If a passive drain is used, then the orientation of the drain must take into account gravity to allow maximum drainage from the exit site. One of the benefits of an active drain is the ability to quantify fluid production, both totals and the trend of production. This measurement can help to guide therapy with regard to when the drain is to be removed. In 1 study in which subcutaneous drains were evaluated in clean wounds, dogs where more likely to develop a seroma after the closed suction drain was removed if fluid production was greater than 0.2 mL/kg per hour.[44] One of the reported complications of closed suction active drains is postoperative hemorrhage owing to disruption of blood clots[45] (**Fig. 2**).

BANDAGING

Before applying the contact layer the skin surrounding the wound should be clean and dry. For bandages on the limbs, stirrups are often used and are thought to prevent slipping of the bandage. Stirrups are made by placing 1-inch white medical tape one-third of the length of the leg on opposing sides and extending equal distance past the digits. Once the contact layer and intermediate layers are placed as described, the distal

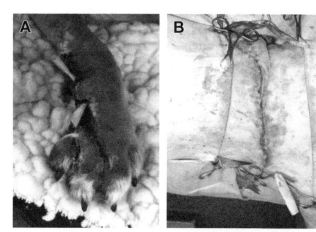

Fig. 2. (*A*) Incorrect placement of a Penrose drain, drain is entering and exiting through the incision and is placed directly beneath the attempted closure. (*B*) Correct placement of a Penrose drain on the lateral abdomen of a dog with the drain exit at least 1 cm from the wound closure and in the most gravity-dependent area of the wound.

ends of the tape are turned 180° and adhered down to the bandage (**Fig. 3**). With regard to the face, neck, proximal limbs, and trunk, bandaging options often have to be more creative. A tie-over bandage can be used to cover wounds of the head, neck, and proximal limbs. To apply a tie-over bandage, stay sutures should be placed in the skin approximately 1 to 2 cm from the edge of the wound with a nonabsorbable monofilament suture of substantial size, such as 2-0 nylon. Layers of the bandage should be placed as described and as appropriate for the character and phase of the wound. The bandage is completed by lacing umbilical tap through the preplaced stay sutures (**Fig. 4**). Alternatively, a circumferential bandage, similar to that described for limbs, can be placed over wounds on the trunk.

Contact Layer

Important considerations for contact layer material are permeability and the absorptive capacity. Bandage material permeability is categorized as occlusive or semiocclusive. An occlusive dressing is meant to create a seal to prevent air and fluid from permeating the layer. Semiocclusive bandages allow for the permeability of fluid and air. Occlusive bandages have the benefit of providing an environment with low oxygen tension that can stimulate macrophage activity, fibroblast proliferation, and angiogenesis. Occlusive bandages also act as a barrier against heat loss, and retaining heat leads to enhanced enzymatic activity. Occlusive bandages have been compared with semiocclusive bandages and certain types have been found to lead to faster wound healing with better cosmetic outcomes.[46,47]

The polymers in hydrocolloid sheets function by absorbing wound exudate to form a gel that is then held to the wound by the scaffold of the dressing. These are most appropriate for mild to moderately exudative wounds and are held in place by additional layers of a semiocclusive bandage.

Heavily exudative wounds may benefit more from either hypertonic saline–soaked bandages or an alginate dressing. Alginate dressings are derived from different types of seaweed and algae, and are available with or without impregnation with silver for its antimicrobial properties. Alginate dressings are applied dry and are very hydrophilic;

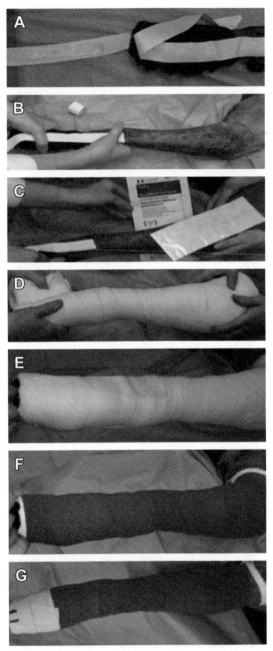

Fig. 3. Appropriate placement of a modified Robert-Jones bandage. (*A*) Placement of 1″ white medical tape stirrups with tongue depressor between strips of tape to prevent adhesion to one another. (*B*) Stirrup tape should extend approximately one-third of the way up the length of the limb. (*C*) Placement of contact layer over incision. (*D*) Intermediate layer of cast padding, overlap of layers approximately 50%. For a true Robert–Jones bandage, either additional layers of cast padding or rolled cotton is used to increase thickness of bandage. (*E*) Intermediate layer gauze cling placed over cast padding with 50% overlap. Stirrups twisted at end and folded back over bandage. (*F*) Outer layer of porous, self-adhesive wrap placed over intermediate layer. Care is taken to leave cast padding at the top and bottom of bandage. (*G*) Porous, cotton elastic cloth tape placed over distal bandage, marker used to mark location of toenails for digits 3 and 4 to monitor to spreading/swelling.

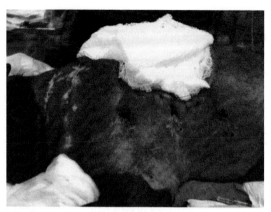

Fig. 4. Tie-over bandage placed on the dorsum of a dog. Note nylon stay sutures around periphery of wound. Umbilical tape laced through stay sutures and over lap pads to hold lap pads in place will be placed next.

as with hydrocolloid sheets, these are also held in place with additional layers of semi-occlusive bandage.

More information on various types of contact layers that also provide antimicrobial effects are outlined in the topical antibiotic section, with a summary provided in **Table 3**.

Intermediate and Outer Layers

The intermediate layer holds the contact layer in place; other functions of the intermediate layer are exudate absorption, pressure, support, and reduction of mobility. The most commonly used intermediate layers are cast padding and rolled cotton, depending on the amount of exudate expected.

The outer layer is responsible for creating the pressure of the bandage; it is most often elastic. The elasticity functions to decrease dead space and fluid accumulation as well as provide support for the wound edges and underlying bandage material. It is preferable for this layer to be porous to allow for the evaporation of fluid from the wound; conversely, this means that this layer will require protecting when the patient is outside in inclement weather or on wet surfaces. Care must be taken when using bandage material with elastic properties to ensure that the bandage is not placed too tight.

Both the intermediate and outer layers are normally placed circumferentially with a 50% overlap with regard to the previous pass of the material. Limbs are wrapped traditionally from distal to proximal with the toenails of digits 3 and 4 visible to monitor for swelling.

NOVEL TREATMENTS

There is ongoing interest in both the biomedical community as well as homeopathic community to advance wound management. Various bioscaffolds are being investigated in veterinary medicine. The purpose of bioscaffolds is to provide a substrate for extracellular matrix formation. They contain growth factors and collagen that should promote matrix deposition, angiogenesis, and epithelialization. Bioscaffolds have been shown to be more useful in chronic as opposed to acute wounds and in fact may be detrimental in acute wound healing (eg, porcine small intestine

Table 3
Common contact layer options, indications, objectives

Contact Layer	Indications	Objectives
Adherent dressings		
Wet–dry or dry–dry	Questionable if ever; potentially inflammatory phase	Absorbs exudate, nonselective debridement; change at least daily
Hyperosmotic agents		
Hypertonic saline	Inflammatory/debridement phases in infected wounds	Desiccates bacteria (antibacterial), nonselective debridement, increases perfusion by decreasing edema; change every 1–3 d
Sugar	Inflammatory to early repair phase	Desiccates bacteria (antibacterial), may provide nutrient source; change at least daily
Honey	Inflammatory to early repair phase	Produces H_2O_2, desiccates bacteria, low pH, inhibin contact (antimicrobial), enhances granulation tissue and epithelialization and reduces edema; change every 1–7 d
Semiocclusive–occlusive nonadherent dressings		
Alginate	Late inflammatory to early repair phase, wound with heavy exudate	Gel forms under pad by absorbing exudate, which keeps a moist environment, Not for use over exposed tendon, bone or necrotic tissue; change every 5–7 d
Petroleum impregnated	Early repair phase	Increases wound contraction; change every 1–3 d
Hydrocolloid	Early repair phase, over healthy granulation tissue with contraction and relatively little exudate. Do not use in infected wounds.	Increases epithelialization, use until granulation tissue covers wound but then may promote excessive granulation tissue; change every 2–3 d
Hydrogel	Inflammatory to repair phase dry wounds with minimal exudate	Absorbs fluid to keep wound moist, use until granulation tissue covers wound but then may promote excessive granulation tissue; can be used to deliver topicals; change every 4–7 d
Perforated polyester film with cotton	Early to mid repair phase, little exudate or over sutured incisions	Increases wound contraction, absorbs exudate; change every 1–3 d
Other		
Triple antibiotic ointment	Inflammatory phase	Reduces surface bacteria load
Silver impregnated	Inflammatory to repair phase, infected wounds	Bactericidal; change every 3–4 d

submucosa).[48,49] Although not a scaffold, platelet-rich plasma may be useful in large or chronic wounds by stimulating healing by the addition of growth factors.[50] Some of the other areas of ongoing research and interest include the use of turmeric,[51,52] milk thistle (*Silybum marianum*),[53] and extracorporeal shockwave therapy,[54] among many others. As with many of our current wound treatment modalities, much of the research is based on case reports and retrospective reviews. Randomized, controlled trials are lacking for both novel treatments and many of the more traditional options.

SUMMARY

Wound care is a complex topic that requires an understanding of normal wound healing, causes of delays of wound healing, and knowledge of the management of wounds. Every wound must be treated as an individual with regard to cause, chronicity, location, and level of microbial contamination, as well as a multitude of patient factors that affect wound healing. Knowledge regarding the types of wound care products available and when NPWT and drain placement is appropriate can improve outcomes with wound healing. Alternatively, use of products at inappropriate phases of healing can cause delays in healing. As a wound progresses through the phases of healing, the management of a wound and the bandage material used must evolve.

REFERENCES

1. Harding KG, Morris HL, Patel GK. Science, medicine and the future: healing chronic wounds. BMJ 2002;324:160–3.
2. Teller P, White TK. The physiology of wound healing: injury through maturation. Surg Clin North Am 2009;89:599–610.
3. Enoch S, Grey JE, Harding KG. Recent advances and emerging treatments. BMJ 2006;332:962–5.
4. Tobias KM, Johnston SA. Veterinary surgery: small animal. St Louis (MO): Elsevier/Saunders; 2012.
5. Singer AJ, Clark RAF. Cutaneous wound healing. N Engl J Med 1999;341:738–46.
6. Fossum TW. Small animal surgery. 3rd edition. St Louis (MO): Mosby Elsevier; 2007.
7. Orgill D, Demling RH. Current concepts and approaches to wound healing. Crit Care Med 1988;16:899–908.
8. Kirby JP, Mazuski JE. Prevention of surgical site infection. Surg Clin North Am 2009;89:365–89, viii.
9. Horan TC, Andrus M, Dudeck MA. CDC/NHSN surveillance definition of health care–associated infection and criteria for specific types of infections in the acute care setting. Am J Infect Control 2008;36:309–32.
10. Turk R, Singh A, Weese JS. Prospective surgical site infection surveillance in dogs. Vet Surg 2015;44:2–8.
11. Alexander JW, Solomkin JS, Edwards MJ. Updated recommendations for control of surgical site infections. Ann Surg 2011;253:1082–93.
12. Anderson D, Podgorny K, Berríos-Torres SI, et al. Strategies to prevent surgical site infections in Acute Care Hospitals: 2014 update. Infect Control Hosp Epidemiol 2014;35:605–27.
13. Sebastian S. Does preoperative scalp shaving result in fewer postoperative wound infections when compared with no scalp shaving? A systematic review. J Neurosci Nurs 2012;44:149–56.
14. Pavletic MM. Atlas of small animal wound management and reconstructive surgery. 3rd edition. Ames (IA): Wiley-Blackwell; 2012.

15. Winkler KP. Factors that interfere with wound healing, the Merck veterinary manual. Whitehouse Station (NJ): Merck Sharp & Dohme Corp; 2012. Available at: http://www.merckmanuals.com/vet/emergency_medicine_and_critical_care/wound_management/factors_that_interfere_with_wound_healing.html.

16. Perez-Tamayo R, Ihnen M. The effect of methionine in experimental wound healing; a morphologic study. Am J Pathol 1953;29:233–49.

17. Blomme EA, Chinn KS, Hardy MM, et al. Selective cyclooxygenase-2 inhibition does not affect the healing of cutaneous full-thickness incisional wounds in SKH-1 mice. Br J Dermatol 2003;148:211–23.

18. Stephens FO, Hunt TK, Jawetz E, et al. Effect of cortisone and vitamin A on wound infection. Am J Surg 1971;121:569–71.

19. Laing EJ. Problems in wound healing associated with chemotherapy and radiation therapy. Probl Vet Med 1990;2:433–41.

20. Amsellem P. Complications of reconstructive surgery in companion animals. Vet Clin North Am Small Anim Pract 2011;41:995–1006.

21. Tucker CB, Mintline EM, Banuelos J, et al. Pain sensitivity and healing of hot-iron cattle brands. J Anim Sci 2014;92:5674–82.

22. Costa FL, Tiussi LD, Nascimento MS, et al. Diclofenac topical gel in excisional wounds maintain heal quality and reduce phlogistic signals. Acta Cir Bras 2014;29:328–33.

23. Nicholson M, Beal M, Shofer F, et al. Epidemiologic evaluation of postoperative wound infection in clean-contaminated wounds: a retrospective study of 239 dogs and cats. Vet Surg 2002;31:577–81.

24. Seguin B, McDonald DE, Kent MS, et al. Tolerance of cutaneous or mucosal flaps placed into a radiation therapy field in dogs. Vet Surg 2005;34:214–22.

25. Bohling MW, Henderson RA, Swaim SF, et al. Comparison of the role of the subcutaneous tissues in cutaneous wound healing in the dog and cat. Vet Surg 2006; 35:3–14.

26. Bohling MW, Henderson RA, Swaim SF, et al. Cutaneous wound healing in the cat: a macroscopic description and comparison with cutaneous wound healing in the dog. Vet Surg 2004;33:579–87.

27. Bohling MW, Henderson RA. Differences in cutaneous wound healing between dogs and cats. Vet Clin North Am Small Anim Pract 2006;36:687–92.

28. Dire DJ, Welsh AP. A comparison of wound irrigation solutions used in the emergency department. Ann Emerg Med 1990;19:704–8.

29. Barnes S, Spencer M, Graham D, et al. Surgical wound irrigation: a call for evidence-based standardization of practice. Am J Infect Control 2014;42:525–9.

30. Liptak JM. An overview of the topical management of wounds. Aust Vet J 1997; 75:408–13.

31. Gall TT, Monnet E. Evaluation of fluid pressures of common wound-flushing techniques. Am J Vet Res 2010;71:1384–6.

32. Buffa EA, Lubbe AM, Verstraete FJ, et al. The effects of wound lavage solutions on canine fibroblasts: an in vitro study. Vet Surg 1997;26:460–6.

33. Fernandez R, Griffiths R. Water for wound cleansing. Cochrane Database Syst Rev 2012;(2):CD003861.

34. Jones G, Wall R. Maggot-therapy in veterinary medicine. Res Vet Sci 2008;85: 394–8.

35. Barie PS, Eachempati SR. Surgical site infections. Surg Clin North Am 2005;85: 1115–35, viii–ix.

36. Malic C, Verchere C, Arneja JS. Inpatient silver sulphadiazine versus outpatient nanocrystalline silver models of care for pediatric scald burns: a value analysis. Can J Plast Surg 2014;22:99–102.
37. Mandal MD, Mandal S. Honey: its medicinal property and antibacterial activity. Asian Pac J Trop Biomed 2011;1:154–60.
38. Demaria M, Stanley BJ, Hauptman JG, et al. Effects of negative pressure wound therapy on healing of open wounds in dogs. Vet Surg 2011;40:658–69.
39. Nolff MC, Fehr M, Bolling A, et al. Negative pressure wound therapy, silver coated foam dressing and conventional bandages in open wound treatment in dogs. A retrospective comparison of 50 paired cases. Vet Comp Orthop Traumatol 2015; 28:30–8.
40. Or M, Van Goethem B, Polis I, et al. Pedicle digital pad transfer and negative pressure wound therapy for reconstruction of the weight-bearing surface after complete digital loss in a dog. Vet Comp Orthop Traumatol 2014;28:140–4.
41. Stanley BJ, Pitt KA, Weder CD, et al. Effects of negative pressure wound therapy on healing of free full-thickness skin grafts in dogs. Vet Surg 2013;42:511–22.
42. Pitt KA, Stanley BJ. Negative pressure wound therapy: experience in 45 dogs. Vet Surg 2014;43:380–7.
43. Ogeer-Gyles JS, Mathews KA, Boerlin P. Nosocomial infections and antimicrobial resistance in critical care medicine. J Vet Emerg Crit Care 2006;16:1–18.
44. Shaver SL, Hunt GB, Kidd SW. Evaluation of fluid production and seroma formation after placement of closed suction drains in clean subcutaneous surgical wounds of dogs: 77 cases (2005-2012). J Am Vet Med Assoc 2014;245:211–5.
45. Lynch AM, Bound NJ, Halfacree ZJ, et al. Postoperative haemorrhage associated with active suction drains in two dogs. J Small Anim Pract 2011;52:172–4.
46. Morgan PW, Binnington AG, Miller CW, et al. The effect of occlusive and semi-occlusive dressings on the healing of acute full-thickness skin wounds on the forelimbs of dogs. Vet Surg 1994;23:494–502.
47. Ramsey DT, Pope ER, Wagner-Mann C, et al. Effects of three occlusive dressing materials on healing of full-thickness skin wounds in dogs. Am J Vet Res 1995;56: 941–9.
48. Schallberger SP, Stanley BJ, Hauptman JG, et al. Effect of porcine small intestinal submucosa on acute full-thickness wounds in dogs. Vet Surg 2008;37:515–24.
49. Winkler JT, Swaim SF, Sartin EA, et al. The effect of a porcine-derived small intestinal submucosa product on wounds with exposed bone in dogs. Vet Surg 2002; 31:541–51.
50. Kim JH, Park C, Park HM. Curative effect of autologous platelet-rich plasma on a large cutaneous lesion in a dog. Vet Dermatol 2009;20:123–6.
51. Akbik D, Ghadiri M, Chrzanowski W, et al. Curcumin as a wound healing agent. Life Sci 2014;116:1–7.
52. Gong C, Wu Q, Wang Y, et al. A biodegradable hydrogel system containing curcumin encapsulated in micelles for cutaneous wound healing. Biomaterials 2013; 34:6377–87.
53. Sharifi R, Pasalar P, Kamalinejad M, et al. The effect of silymarin (Silybum marianum) on human skin fibroblasts in an in vitro wound healing model. Pharm Biol 2013;51:298–303.
54. Link KA, Koenig JB, Silveira A, et al. Effect of unfocused extracorporeal shock wave therapy on growth factor gene expression in wounds and intact skin of horses. Am J Vet Res 2013;74:324–32.

Peri-Surgical Nutrition

Perspectives and Perceptions

Christopher W. Frye, DVM, April E. Blong, DVM, Joseph J. Wakshlag, PhD, DVM*

KEYWORDS

- Nutrition • Immunonutrition • Arginine • Omega-3 fatty acids • Perioperative

KEY POINTS

- The enteral route is always preferred over the parenteral route because of the decreased infection complication rates.
- Enteral nutrition using immunomodulating agents, such as omega-3 fatty acids, arginine, and glutamine, may decrease infectious complication rates and shorten hospital stays based on human meta-analysis data.
- Esophagostomy and gastrostomy tubes are preferred tubes for long-term nutritional management.
- When instituting enteral or parenteral support, monitoring for refeeding is suggested, particularly after prolonged anorexia.

NUTRITION IN HOSPITALIZED SURGICAL PATIENTS

For many years medicine has recognized that deficiencies in essential nutrients and malnutrition may compromise healing and outcomes in hospitalized patients. In the last 30 years, a movement has been initiated to investigate the supplementation of nutritional elements that may provide an impact extending beyond the provision of nutrition alone, providing discrete therapeutic functions. The provision of specific nutrients in an attempt to beneficially modulate the immune system for certain injuries or disease states has been coined *immunonutrition*. This movement has not been translated particularly well to veterinary medicine because of the paucity of literature and the unique demands of dogs and cats, which make assimilation of the current information difficult, yet worth discussing. One dogma that has translated well to veterinary medicine is the idea that the gastrointestinal (GI) system, when functional, is the preferred route of nutrient administration. In veterinary medicine, the use of parenteral

The authors have nothing to disclose.
Department of Clinical Sciences, Cornell University College of Veterinary Medicine, 930 Campus Road, Ithaca, NY 14853, USA
* Corresponding author.
E-mail address: jw37@cornell.edu

approaches remains in its infancy: there are few prospective veterinary clinical trials and a paucity of veterinary literature showing any substantial benefits other than in severely malnourished patients. This review focuses on the idea of immunonutrition in human medicine and its possible use in veterinary medicine, elaborates on the current options for and understanding of enteral support in our veterinary patients, and provides a cursory guideline into utilization of parenteral nutrition (PN) in surgical patients when deemed necessary.

ENTERAL SUPPORT AND IMMUNONUTRITION

The provision of nutrients with potential immune-modulating effects at either physiologic or supraphysiologic level may be used as a treatment or for prevention of disease.[1,2] These immunomodulating diets (IMDs) typically consist of a combination of nutrients that may include arginine, glutamine, omega-3 fatty acids (n-3 FAs), antioxidants, and nucleotides. Most recently, the term *pharmaconutrition* has been used when discussing the optimal nutrient profile for a specific patient's needs; however, defining this ideal profile currently remains an intangible goal, particularly in veterinary medicine.[3] Some of the discordance within the literature addressing IMD effects may be attributed to applying the same ingredient formula to a heterogeneous population.[4] Regardless, sufficient evidence exists supporting the use of immunonutrition in hospitalized patients for wound healing, elective GI surgeries, and critical or intensive care situations. The proposed mechanisms behind the most commonly used immune modulating nutrients and a brief review of some of the more pertinent literature addressing IMDs and their clinical outcomes for elective surgery and critical care patients are outlined further.

Arginine

Arginine is an amino acid that may be synthesized de novo in humans from citrulline by the kidney tubule epithelium[5] and plays a major role in the urea cycle.[1] Rapid depletion in times of severe stress and other circumstances that lead to a catabolic state may make arginine a "conditionally essential amino acid in humans,"[2] and it is known that arginine is essential in the diet of cats and dogs.[6–8] Arginine has specific functions in both acute and chronic phases of healing. It contributes to protein synthesis, cellular proliferation and differentiation, possesses antimicrobial effects and vascular effects, mediates progression of the immune response, increases insulin sensitivity, and influences growth factor and growth hormone signaling.[1–3,5,9]

Arginine acts through several different pathways to influence the immune system, as it is a precursor to proline, nitric oxide (NO), and ornithine. Inducible NO synthase (iNOS) is an enzyme that is upregulated during periods of T-helper 1 (Th1) cytokine response (influenced by interleukin 1 [IL-1], tumor necrosis factor [TNF]-α, interferon-γ, or other stimuli such as lipopolysaccharide) and converts arginine to NO.[9–11] NO provides direct antimicrobial activity through the oxidative burst and has vascular effects that allow leukocyte migration and increased blood flow to the local wound environment during acute injury.[1,12] NO also has several cellular signaling roles and may induce growth factor release (vascular endothelial growth factor and transforming growth factor [TGF]-β) to help transition from the inflammatory to proliferative pathways while promoting cellular protection, keratinocyte proliferation, and angiogenesis.[1,5,11] During a Th2 response, or following a shift from the inflammatory phase to the proliferative phase in normal wound healing, cytokines, such as IL-4, IL-10, IL-13, and TGF-β, are released. These signaling molecules tip the balance from iNOS toward arginase-1–driven enzymatic reactions.[3,10] Arginase-1 competitively reduces arginine available for iNOS while simultaneously forming ornithine and proline. Ornithine may then be used to synthesize polyamines, which act as building blocks for cellular proliferation and growth during wound repair, whereas proline becomes a major component of collagen during scar tissue formation.[1] Arginine, therefore, plays important roles throughout the normal inflammatory, proliferative, and maturation phases of wound healing.

Despite the overwhelming positive literature base for arginine supplementation in wound healing and immune stimulation, a study in dogs using parenteral arginine supplementation given during experimentally induced sepsis found decreased survival caused by cardiovascular complications.[13] Although this study used parenteral arginine, it serves as a reminder that a thorough understanding of the potential benefits and risks are key to proper nutrient utilization. There are no trials in critically ill or surgical veterinary patients to provide dosing guidelines for any IMD components. The only arginine-enriched enteral veterinary diet studied contained arginine at just more than 5% dry matter. The study found marginal benefits in remission and survival time in dogs with stage III lymphoma fed the enriched diet; however, the diet was also enriched in n-3 FA.[14]

Glutamine

Glutamine has also been considered a conditionally essential amino acid that can become deficient during critical illness or GI disorders.[3,4] This amino acid is released in disproportionately high amounts from skeletal muscle during periods of catabolism caused by stress, sepsis, or injury.[3,15] Enterocytes preferably use glutamine as a source of energy, helping to maintain gut integrity and villi architecture and decrease bacterial translocation, and fuels leukocytes within gut-associated lymphoid tissue.[3,4,12] The antioxidant glutathione relies on glutamine for production and, when reduced, may lead to diarrhea, malabsorption, mucosal degradation, and failure to thrive.[3] Glutamine dampens the Th1 inflammatory response by reducing IL-6, TNF-α, and nuclear factor kappa beta (NF-κB) of activated B cells following sepsis and helps protect vital organs during ischemia reperfusion and sepsis.[3,4,9,16] In addition, glutamine helps to induce heat shock proteins, which act as chaperones for denatured proteins, to provide cellular protection from inflammatory injury.[2,9,17] Plasma arginine levels may be increased through enzymatic production from glutamine.[9] Although an increased demand for glutamine has been demonstrated postoperatively, there remains discordance in the literature regarding the benefits of glutamine supplementation in reducing surgical morbidity.[15,18] In veterinary patients, the utilization of glutamine may have some validity; however, the use of high quantities of digestible protein often surpasses human enteral formulas. This increased protein consumption in veterinary patients raises questions relating to the utility of amino acid supplementation in small animal surgical patients as a means of providing and immune-modulating benefits when enteral nutrition is initiated.

Omega-3 Fatty Acids

The n-3 FAs mediate the inflammatory response either directly or indirectly. They inactivate NF-κB signal transduction pathways and reduce inflammatory cytokine TNF-α production by lipopolysaccharide-induced macrophages.[2,19] The n-3 FAs, in particular eicosapentaenoic acid and docosahexaenoic acid, will displace omega-6 FAs (n-6 FAs), such as arachidonic acid from cell membranes. When these n-3 FAs are liberated from the plasma membranes and acted on by lipoxygenase and cyclooxygenase enzymes, they produce inert or less inflammatory eicosanoids compared with n-6 FAs, thereby reducing inflammation.[2,3,19] Lastly, they help produce resolvins and protectins, which might dampen and help resolve the inflammatory response.[3,20] The supplementation of long-chain n-3 FAs does not go without controversy, as some suggest that dampening the inflammatory cascade can lead to immunosuppression. Rodent studies have shown that high concentrations of the n-3 FAs eicosapentaenoic acid and docosahexaenoic acid in the diet prevent a heighted immune response to infectious organisms, potentially worsening the disease process.[21,22] This dampening of the immune response may indicate there is a safe upper limit and optimal dose to modulate, but not hinder the immune response to pathogens.

OTHER POTENTIAL IMMUNONUTRIENTS

Nucleotides are composed of a purine or pyrimidine base on a sugar backbone with one or more phosphate groups. They are components of deoxyribonucleic acid, ribonucleic acid, adenosine triphosphate, and many other cellular intermediates.[3,9] For this reason, nucleotides (supplemented as RNA) have been shown to assist in rapid cell division, such as during an immune response or wound healing.[12,23] Antioxidants or cofactors in the antioxidant or immune response may also possess immunomodulating effects and may include vitamin A, vitamin C, selenium, and zinc.[2,3,9] However, their applications in veterinary patients has not been studied; the replete nature of commercial dog and cat foods designed for recovery make the application difficult to assimilate into surgical veterinary practices.

The Impact of Immunonutrition in Human Patients

Elective surgery patients

Many studies and meta-analyses have recently been conducted regarding perioperative immunonutrition for elective GI, head and neck, and cardiac surgery, often demonstrating decreased length of hospital stay (LOS), decreased concentrations of inflammatory mediators, better gut microprofusion, and fewer postoperative complications, such as infection or dehiscence.[12,20,23–29] Most of this research has been oriented around elective GI surgeries with enteral IMDs.[18] Surgery is a traumatic insult that results in a period of immunosuppression within a patient population that may already have a weakened immune system related to being malnourished and other comorbidities.[18,19,30,31] GI surgery alone results in decreased gut microprofusion, altered gut mucosal structure, increased risk of bacterial and endotoxin translocation, and upregulation of arginase-1 through a Th2 inflammatory response. This upregulation inhibits NO production and limits arginine as a substrate for normal T-lymphocyte function.[25,26] When examining patients undergoing colorectal surgeries without nutritional deficiencies, immunonutrition still led to better outcomes.[24] This research indicates that nutrient supplementation has pharmaceutical effects beyond nutrient repletion, hence, the term *pharmaconutrition*.

Certain combinations of immunonutrients are more effective than those given alone, and some studies have demonstrated a synergism between arginine and n-3 FAs.[16,24,25,31] For example, arginine supplementation with n3-FAs has been shown to upregulate NO production, decrease bacterial translocation, and increase local gut perfusion.[18,19] However, arginine alone may still be beneficial to many patients, as administration of NO inhibitors has been shown to limit the protective effects of arginine within the gut.[18,32]

The exact timing, quantity, and composition of immunonutrients have yet to be determined. Various combinations and amounts of nutrients are available in commercial IMDs, which are typically supplemented with 2 or more of the following ingredients: arginine, n-3 FAs, nucleotides, glutamine, and antioxidants.[25,33] Drover and colleagues[25] conducted the largest systematic review on perioperative immunonutrition in elective surgery with 35 randomized controlled trials (RCTs) and more than 3000 patients. They were able to compare different commercial formulations and found that patients that received Impact (Nestle Health Science, Florham Park, NJ, USA) had significant reductions in postoperative complications, which was not seen with other formulas. Impact was the only formulation that included nucleotides and lacked supplemental glutamine. Drover and colleagues[25] also found that the beneficial effects of perioperative nutrition were superior to either preoperative or postoperative nutrition alone. Most other meta-analyses and systematic reviews find that IMDs given preoperatively and perioperatively are superior to those administered postoperatively; however, postoperative immunonutrition still results in better clinical outcomes than isocaloric traditional nutritional approaches.[18,23,34,35]

These studies found better results with earlier intervention, which may be attributable to overcoming the delay in nutrient uptake by affected tissues as well as an inevitable reduction in postoperative feeding volume that impedes appropriate caloric and nutritional uptake.[15,36] Giger and colleagues[26] studied the timing of perioperative versus postoperative nutrition in an RCT for major elective abdominal surgery. Perioperative IMDs significantly reduced systemic inflammation and postoperative complications compared with postoperative IMDs alone. In a systematic review by Zhang and colleagues,[35] perioperative IMDs were found to decrease noninfectious complications more than preoperative or postoperative administration alone. It seems that perioperative nutrition has greater benefits than postoperative nutrition in reducing morbidity (especially infectious complications) and LOS, but no effect on mortality has been shown.

Critically ill patients

Within critically ill patient populations, there remains much discordance among various studies and meta-analyses regarding the use of immunonutrition; however, enteral nutrition, whenever possible, seems superior to parenteral nutrition.[30,37–40] A systematic review by Montejo and colleagues[39] found benefits using immunonutrition in 26 relevant studies, showing a decreased infection rate, intensive care unit (ICU) LOS, and ventilator time that depended on the subgroup of patients analyzed. Within these studies, there was no effect on mortality rate or the development of systemic inflammatory response syndrome (SIRS) or acute respiratory distress syndrome (ARDS), similar to elective surgery patients on IMDs. When the patients were divided into subgroups based on the cause of their illness, it was found that trauma patients had a reduction in bacteremia and intra-abdominal infections; surgical patients had reduced wound and urinary tract infections; and burn patients had a reduction in nosocomial pneumonia. ICU patients remained the only group with a decreased LOS.

A systematic review by Marik and Zaloga[41] classified the type of IMD included in the analysis. They found that only fish oil (n-3 FAs) decreased mortality, infection, and LOS in ICU patients with SIRS, sepsis, or ARDS. In addition, it was noted that arginine may be detrimental when added to the fish oil–supplemented diet. Many other studies have indicated that arginine supplementation may be harmful in critically ill patients (especially those experiencing severe SIRS or sepsis) as it upregulates NO to a point that may lead to cardiovascular collapse and increased mortality.[3,13,37,41] Studies showing beneficial effects of IMDs with added arginine were mainly composed of heterogeneous populations of critically ill patients who underwent elective surgical procedures, biasing the results.[42,43] Glutamine is similarly controversial in critically ill populations, often having no influence or even adverse consequences.[18,30,37,40] However, in contrast to specific amino acids, n-3 FA supplementation alone may have substantial benefits, including a reduction in both mortality and morbidity.[37,38,44,45]

Another major factor beyond patient selection and IMD choice is the timing of supplementation. In critical patients, earlier supplementation may be more beneficial, perhaps intervening before the inflammatory response reaches a stage impervious to nutritional support.[30,40,44] Pontes-Arruda and colleagues[44] provided enteral eicosapentaenoic acid and γ-linolenic acid (an n-6 FA with antiinflammatory properties) to 106 eligible patients who were septic, but had yet to develop multiorgan dysfunction syndrome and compared this with an isocaloric, isonitrogenous control diet without added lipids in an RCT. This study found significant reductions in development of severe sepsis or septic shock (26% vs 51%, $P = .0217$). An earlier meta-analysis by the same investigators[45] found supplementation of n-3 FAs with γ-linolenic acid beneficial for patients with ARDS. Within that study there was a significant reduction in mortality, development of multiorgan dysfunction syndrome, ventilator days, and length of ICU stay. In contrast, another study demonstrated n-3 FA supplementation had no effect on decreasing ventilator days; however, this study included a more heterogeneous patient population.[46]

The use of IMDs in critically ill patients remains controversial depending on the population treated, timing of the treatment, and the dose and composition of the supplement. Although both benefits and detriments to IMDs have been shown, almost all investigators tend to concur that enteral feeding is superior to parenteral administration when available. Clearly, further studies and meta-analyses are warranted.

Immunonutrition in Veterinary Patients

Literature relating to the use of perioperative immunonutrition in small animals is relatively sparse. A single, double-blind, randomized, placebo-controlled study assessed the effects of a diet supplemented with fish oil (n-3 FAs) and arginine on the survival time of dogs with lymphoma that were treated with doxorubricin.[14] The study diet contained an n-6:3 FA ratio of 0.3:1% and 5.54% arginine on a dry-matter basis. Dogs fed the study diet had a slightly longer mean disease-free interval and survival time, but this was only significant in patients with stage IIIa disease. The study included both dogs with stage IIIa and IVa lymphoma. Unfortunately, the study did not specify how the stages were distributed across the groups, as a significantly decreased median survival time and disease-free interval was seen in the dogs with stage IV disease.

An experimental study assessing the effect of n-3 FAs on wound healing in beagles revealed that a 4-day-old wound in dogs fed a diet with a normal n-6:3 FA ratio of 5.3:1 had lower levels of arachidonic acid/eicosapentaenoic acid in wounded tissue.[47] However, no histopathologic differences could be found.

An observational study in critically ill dogs documented lower plasma levels of several amino acids relative to healthy control dogs, including alanine, arginine, methionine, serine, citrulline, glycine, and proline.[48] Survivors had higher levels of arginine, isoleucine, leucine, serine, valine, and total branched-chain amino acids. Because this was an observational study, the question of whether or not supplementing these amino acids can improve outcomes in veterinary ICU patients remains unanswered.

Despite this paucity of veterinary literature, the availability of human commercially available immunonutrition diets (ie, Impact) certainly begs the questions of whether or not these products would be suitable for veterinary use and if they would clinically influence relevant outcome measures in patients. Although these diets may be used short-term in hospitalized dogs (as they meet the National Research Council's recommended nutrients on a kilocalorie basis for nearly all nutrients), the unique metabolism of cats precludes their extended use in feline patients.

Assisted Enteral Nutrition

The patients who are likely to benefit most from nutritional supplementation are invariably the ones that will not voluntarily eat. Fortunately, there are several potential intervention options, including pharmacotherapy, syringe feeding, nasogastric/nasoesophageal tubes, esophagostomy tubes, gastrostomy tubes (G tubes), and jejunostomy tubes (J tubes).

Pharmacotherapy treatments to increase appetite are often considered. In the authors' experience, appetite stimulants are typically not successful in critically ill patients, but do tend to help the patients who are not eating because of stress or mild illness. Benzodiazepines (midazolam or diazepam) given intravenously at low doses, 0.05 to 0.1 mg/kg, can stimulate appetites in some animals.[49] Patients should be monitored closely to ensure that sedation from these medications does not preclude a tolerance to oral diet intake. Such treatment is subjectively more successful in cats than dogs. In dogs, the use of propofol at 1 to 3 mg/kg body weight has been shown to induce transient hyperphagia; such effects may be used in a diagnostic manner to examine the tolerance of oral feeding when nausea and emesis are suspect.[50] Mirtazapine is a tetracyclic antidepressant with effects at serotonergic neurons that result in increased appetite. The dosage for cats is 3.75 mg per cat once every 3 days, whereas the suggested dosage for dogs is 0.3 mg/kg once daily.[49,51]

Syringe or assisted/force feeding is rarely indicated and is never appropriate for more than a couple feedings. It is often stressful, disliked by patients, and can occasionally cause oral trauma. The amount of nutrition that can be supplied through this method is limited, making it difficult to meet the resting energy requirement (RER) of a patient. Force feeding can also lead to food aversion causing a patient, who would otherwise eat, to refuse the appropriate diet. It is contraindicated in any patient with orofacial trauma, a decreased ability to swallow, or a reduced gag reflex.

A *nasogastric or nasoesophageal* tube is an excellent short-term intervention for many ICU or postsurgical patients. These tubes are available in a variety of styles, lengths, and with or without weighted tips to facilitate passage into the stomach. Softer, more flexible tubes typically provide greater patient comfort. Whether to place the tube in the esophagus or the stomach is somewhat patient dependent. Tubes that do not pass through the lower esophageal sphincter may have less risk of associated gastroesophageal reflux. However, by passing the tube into the stomach, measuring pH and quantity of gastric contents is possible.[52] This possibility may be particularly useful in a patient with altered GI motility or regurgitating/vomiting causing gastric overdistention. Methods for placing these tubes can be referenced from a variety of sources.[53–55] Regardless of the position chosen, placement should be confirmed radiographically before initiating feeding to avoid inadvertently administering food into the airway. Feeding tubes can also coil or turn on themselves during placement or after a vomiting episode. If the esophagus is to be the final position, the distal tip of the tube should be positioned between the base of the heart and the diaphragm.[55] For tubes that end in the stomach, it is important to be sure that the tube stoma is in the stomach to allow for aspiration of gastric contents. This placement is particularly important for tubes with weighted ends as the actual opening can be a few centimeters from the distal end of the tube. Excessive lengths of tube should not be left in the stomach as it is possible for the tube end to migrate out of the stomach into the duodenum or become knotted or kinked. Care should be taken to ensure the tube remains appropriately positioned after vomiting or regurgitation to ensure tube eversion has not occurred before further feeding is carried out. Because of the small diameter typically used (usually 5–12 F) and the long tube length, a liquid diet is typically necessary. Tubes that are 10 to 12 F or larger can often tolerate a well-blended diet that is smooth in consistency. Crushed and well-dissolved pills or liquid oral medications may also be given through these larger tubes.

Absolute contraindications for these types of tubes are few. Persistent vomiting or regurgitation may make these tubes difficult to keep appropriately placed; many patients experience some discomfort and will try to remove them, necessitating an Elizabethan collar. These tubes frequently cause rhinitis, sinusitis, and dacryocystitis. Care should be taken in patients if the nasal passages are already occluded or there is preexisting respiratory distress as further occluding the nares can worsen or cause the development of respiratory distress.[52,55] This point is particularly true in cats as they often do not tolerate having both nares occluded. Patients who are prone to bleeding may not be good candidates for nasal tube placement as any bleeding induced during placement may be difficult to control. Animals who may have elevated intracranial pressure or are at risk for changes in intracranial pressure may also not be good candidates for nasal tube placement. Sneezing is often stimulated during placement and can cause intracranial pressure to spike.[56] A nasoesophageal tube is contraindicated in patients with a reduced gag reflex, inability to protect their airway, esophageal dysmotility, or megaesophagus; however, nasogastric tubes can be used cautiously. If there is esophageal trauma or stricture, then other feeding tubes should be considered. Most patients will require some amount of sedation to place these tubes; although for most ill patients, only a mild sedative, such as butorphanol, is necessary.

Esophagostomy tubes can be used for short- or long-term use. Not only are they useful for feeding but medications can also be administered. For owners with mobility difficulties or in fractious patients (cats most commonly), an esophageal tube for medication administration may allow an owner to treat a patient that could not otherwise be treated. Although trained personnel can place them rapidly, brief anesthesia is still required. These tubes can be used as soon as patients are recovered from anesthesia and able to adequately protect their airway. Silicone or polyurethane tubes should be used if the tube is needed for more than a couple of weeks, as other types of tubes can become brittle and crack. Most cats will tolerate a 14-F tube, and dogs can have an 18-F tube or larger. These larger bore tubes have the advantage of allowing almost any blended diet to be administered as well as oral medications. Potential complications apart from anesthesia include stoma infection or cellulitis, rarely esophageal stricture at the stoma site, and damage to cervical nerves or vascular structures during placement.[52,55,57] The tube can be placed on either side of the neck; however, because of the anatomic esophageal course, the left side becomes the preferred insertion site.[58] The main contraindications for an esophagostomy tube are esophageal disease or cervical trauma, and vomiting can still potentially cause the tube to evert similar to nasoesophageal or nasogastric tubes.

If feeding tube support is likely to be needed long-term (months to years), a G tube is likely a better option. G tubes can be placed using a variety of methods that are covered elsewhere.[57,58] They are typically large in diameter (18 F or larger), accommodating most diet options and medications. In patients undergoing abdominal surgery who are already acutely or chronically ill, preemptive G-tube placement at the initial time of surgery should be considered to prevent a second anesthesia solely for feeding tube placement. In patients not undergoing surgery, percutaneous endoscopic gastrostomy (PEG) tube placement is typically preferred. However, when compared with surgically placed G tubes, PEG tubes have higher complication rates related to stoma formation, infection, and septic peritonitis.[59] All G tubes require an adhesion to form around the stoma site joining the stomach to the body wall to prevent leakage of gastric contents into the peritoneum resulting in potentially catastrophic peritonitis and sepsis. This adhesion around the stoma develops in 7 to 10 days and potentially longer in patients with immunosuppression or delayed wound healing.[57] To ensure a fibrous seal has occurred before feeding, the first feeding is typically delayed for 12 to 24 hours after tube placement. In patients with potential healing deficits or poor apposition of the stomach to the body wall (obesity, large-breed dogs, presence of ascites), surgical tube placement with pexy will likely carry less risk.[57]

Similar to nasogastric tubes, these tubes also allow for assessment of gastric residual volumes, gastric decompression, and monitoring of gastric pH. The main contraindication for G-tube placement is primary gastric disease. As with any enteral feeding, it should be used cautiously in animals with an impaired gag reflex or mentation. A low-profile tube can be exchanged for the traditional G tube once adequate stoma adhesion has occurred.

J tubes have the potential advantage of bypassing the proximal duodenum and all adoral structures. This advantage reduces the likelihood of food refluxing back into the stomach or esophagus; however, it will not stop normal gastric secretions and their potential reflux. Tube placement is most often performed surgically with the intestine being sutured to the abdominal wall to facilitate stoma formation; however, methods to feed a J tube through a G tube using endoscopic techniques have also been described.[60] Cats and small dogs will typically tolerate a 5-F tube, whereas in larger dogs an 8-F tube can be used; small tube diameter necessitates feeding a liquid diet.[58] The main contraindication to J-tube placement is a distal intestinal obstruction. Accidental dislodgement or tube migration is a significant complication with J tubes.[57] Other potential complications include leakage from the enterostomy site causing peritonitis, catheter perforation of the intestine, and leakage of contents subcutaneously leading to necrosis, infection, and cellulitis.[52,55,57] These tubes can be used immediately after placement. If placed surgically, the placement of sutures to pexy the intestine to the body wall can reduce the chances of peritonitis if the tube is inadvertently removed.[57] Regardless of the surgical technique used, it is advisable to leave the tube in place for at least 5 to 7 days to allow for adequate adhesion formation.[58]

The intestinal tract is used to chyme being slowly released from the stomach over time and does not have a mechanism for dealing with large bolus feedings. Therefore, J-tube feeding should be performed via constant rate infusion. As a J tube will bypass the duodenum, there are concerns that a lack of appropriate pancreatic enzymes will lead to incomplete protein, fat, and carbohydrate digestion in typical enteral feeds. Therefore, it is often best to use elemental diets, such as Vivonex Plus (Nestle Health Science, Florham Park, NJ, USA), to ensure absorption of amino acids, fatty acids, and simple carbohydrates. However, many clinicians use normal liquid enteral diets with success; but if diarrhea is present, conversion to an elemental diet may be beneficial. In cats, there may be few options as the typical elemental diets used are designed for human consumption and are often insufficient in protein, taurine, and selected vitamins.

With any enteral approach used, the RER should be met in perioperative patients. Some have advocated an illness energy requirement that increases the energy provided to more than the RER, but these typically do not apply to surgical or hospitalized patients.[55] The only time that more calories than the RER may be necessary is after acute trauma, burns, certain critically ill patients, and degloving injuries whereby extreme losses of proteinaceous fluids may lead to increased energy and protein demands. Often surgical patients have inappetence or are anorexic for several days before surgery; therefore, when refeeding these patients, a gradual approach is adopted and is outlined in **Box 1**. This gradual reintroduction to food is thought to decrease the potential for refeeding syndrome (hyperglycemia, hypokalemia, and hypophosphatemia) that can occur with aggressive reintroduction of food, which occurs more frequently in cats.[61]

Box 1
Small animal enteral nutrition work sheet

Actual body weight: _____*kg; Ideal body weight:* _____*kg*

1. RER: 70 (kg body weight)$^{0.75}$ = _____kcal/d
   OR
   Illness energy requirement: 1.0–1.5 × RER = _____kcal/d (ie, trauma, burns, and so forth)

2. Product selected

   Product selected_____

   Blended contains _____kcal/mL

   RER _____/_____ kcal/mL= _____mL/d

3. Administration schedule:

   One-third of total requirement on day 1: 0.33 × _____mL/d = _____mL/d

   Two-thirds of total requirement on day 2: 0.67 × _____mL/d = _____mL/d

   Total requirement on day 3 = _____mL/d

4. Feeding schedule: divide total volume into 4 to 6 feedings per day

   a. Day 1 total volume_____/4 or 6 = _____per feeding per day 1

   b. Day 2 total volume_____/4 or 6 = _____per feeding per day 2

   c. Full volume_____/4 or 6 = _____per feeding per day 3

5. General instructions

   a. Before feeding aspirate the tube (note and record residual volume, if more than 20% of the volume administered previously, return the liquid to the stomach and delay feeding).

   b. Flush the tube with _____mL of warm water (amount will depend on type of tube used).

   c. Administer warmed diet over 5 to 10 minutes. If vomiting occurs, stop the feeding and notify the clinical staff.

   d. Flush the tube with _____mL warm water, recap, and rewrap if necessary.

Parenteral Support

If enteral support is not an option, then PN support should be considered, particularly if the patient is malnourished. In veterinary medicine, we are often hesitant to initiate PN because of the cost and a lack of evidence to support its use for improving hospitalization outcomes or LOS. Much of the veterinary literature is retrospective in nature, primarily examining complication rates.[62–67] Parenteral support can be administered either via a peripheral or central vein. This selection of venous access becomes important when formulating the diet as the final osmolality of peripheral solutions should not exceed 700 mOsm/L (see later discussion). In veterinary patients, particularly cats, the metabolic complication most often encountered is hyperglygemia.[64,65] Mechanical complications are also common (ie, feeding line occlusions, phlebitis, and patient removal). Parenteral support should only be considered when enteral support is not an option because of medical complications; enteral support is considered superior as it prevents transmigration of bacteria to the portal blood and improves the immunologic status of patients.[68]

Parenteral support is not well studied in veterinary medicine, and the relative use and utility of the 3 main substrates (glucose, amino acid, and lipid) differ depending on the source of information.[55,69,70] Glucose and lipid are often used to meet most of the calorie requirements. The precise mixture of these two components will depend on an individual patient's underlying conditions, such as hyperglycemia, hypertriglyceridemia, or ketosis. The parenteral protein requirements for ill cats and dogs is currently unknown, and we can only assume the requirement is similar to healthy animals. Extrapolation from human data suggests that protein turnover may be higher during catabolic illness; in the authors' formulations, is used than typically more protein required. In an elegantly designed study, it was found that provision of approximately 2.3 g of protein per kilogram of body weight supplied as a parenteral amino acid solution is adequate in healthy dogs.[71] This finding suggests that adding 2.5 to 3.0 g/kg of amino acid solution for a dog is likely sufficient and 4 g of protein per kilogram of body weight is often used as a starting point for cats. Amino acids come in several different formulations and strengths (eg, 5.5%, 8.5%, and 10.0%), with and without electrolytes. Amino acids with electrolytes typically provide basal sodium, chloride, magnesium, phosphorus, and potassium requirements when used at 1.5 to 2.5 g/kg body weight of protein; however, these are used less often in veterinary species, particularly in cats whose protein requirement may be higher. When using amino acids with electrolytes, the electrolytes provided should be considered before supplementing additional electrolytes in fluids. **Box 2** describes a typical parenteral feeding program for a cat or dog using a 10% amino acid solution without electrolytes. During the first day of PN, it is typically recommended to provide only half of the calorie requirement, particularly if there has been a history of anorexia. This recommendation is made because of the potential for refeeding syndrome. This recommendation also illustrates the need to assess electrolyte status every 12 to 24 hours for the first 48 to 72 hours when implementing parenteral support.

PN formulation should be done in a laminar flow hood with appropriate aseptic procedures to prevent contamination of solutions. Prior concerns about PN and complications, such as yeast or bacterial contamination or lipid emboli, are not warranted. Recent evidence suggests that in a typical veterinary formulated PN solution, the lipid particles remain well emulsified and no bacterial growth was evident for 3 days following formulation when kept refrigerated.[72] Peripheral PN, with its lower osmolality, is at an increased risk of microbial growth, thus more caution should be taken with these formulations.

The typical osmolality and pH of a PN solution will be far different than plasma osmolality (around 1000–1300 mOsm and pH <7). This high osmolality may be irritating to the vascular endothelium and requires a large central vessel for administration.[70] Such high osmolar solutions cannot be used in a peripheral vein as they may induce thrombophlebitis and is the reason that 5% dextrose is used to dilute peripheral PN solutions rather than the 50% dextrose solution used in central PN formulations.[63,69] Using 5% dextrose creates an osmolality of less than 700 mOsm/L, which is a guideline from human medicine that has been adopted by many veterinary nutritionists.[73] **Box 3** shows typical guidelines for peripheral PN formulation for dogs and cats.[63,69] The addition of B-complex vitamins should also be considered when using PN; however, typically the need for PN is very short lived (2–5 days) postsurgically; therefore, consideration for long-term management is not discussed.

Regardless of the site to be used, it is important to ensure that a PN-dedicated catheter or lumen (in multi-lumen catheters) is used. Drugs should never be coadministered in the PN-dedicated port or line. Avoiding injections, minimizing flushes, and avoiding opening the port or line of this catheter or lumen will reduce the chances

---

Box 2
Small animal total PN formulation sheet

$RER = 70 \ (kg \ body \ weight)^{0.75}$; $RER =$ _____

1. Protein req:

Dogs: 3 g/kg body weight; Cats: 4 g/kg/body weight

  Protein req (g/d) = _____g/kg × body weight kg = _____g/d

  Protein calories (g/d) × 4 kcal/g = _____kcal/d

  Total kilocalories – protein calories = _____nonprotein calories (NPC)

2. NPC

    Dextrose (40%–60%) NPC; _____% × NPC = _____kcal dextrose

    Lipid (40%–60%) NPC; _____% × NPC = _____kcal lipid

3. Volumes of substrates

    8.5% amino acid solution = 0.085 g/mL

    Protein g req _____/0.085 g = _____mL of amino acid solution * one-half volume for day 1_____

    50% dextrose (kcal) _____/1.7 kcal/mL = _____mL of 50% dextrose * one-half volume for day 1_____

    20% lipid (kcal) _____/2.0 kcal/mL = _____mL of 20% lipid * one-half volume for day 1_____

Total volume of TPN solution = _____mL/24 h = _____mL/h * one-half volume for day 1_____ per 24 h = _____

Fluid req _____mL – TPN volume _____mL = remaining fluid req _____mL

Remaining fluid req per 24 hours = _____mL/h of fluids

Abbreviations: NPC, nonprotein calories; req, requirement; TPN, total PN.

---

for microbial colonization. The catheter should be placed using a strict aseptic technique. In human medicine, the use of catheter care packages, which include the use of chlorhexidine antiseptic, sterile gowns, gloves, and full-body draping of the patients, have been shown to reduce the number of catheter-associated blood stream infections associated with the use of central catheters.[74] It is unclear if similar protocols would be beneficial in veterinary medicine. Regardless of the catheter type, the insertion site should be inspected and cleaned every 12 to 24 hours; the vein should be palpated for signs of pain or firmness, which may indicate phlebitis; and the site should be kept clean and dry. If any redness, swelling, discharge at the insertion site, or signs of phlebitis are noted, the catheter should be immediately removed and the tip should be saved for potential bacteriologic culture. The presence of an otherwise unexplainable new fever in a patient should also prompt evaluation of all catheters and their potential replacement.

A central venous catheter terminates in the vena cava (cranial or caudal). This catheter can be introduced into the jugular vein or a longer peripherally inserted central catheter (PICC). Central or PICC catheters may be preferred if multiple lumens, repeated sampling access, or the ability to measure central venous pressures is desired. Patient soiling and cleanliness is particularly important as the limbs are much more likely to be contaminated by urine or feces than the neck. Patients with

---

Box 3
Small animal partial PN formulation sheet

$RER = 70 \ (kg \ body \ weight)^{0.75}$; $RER =$ _____ $\times \ 0.50 =$ _____ partial energy required

1. Nutrient distributions
   a. Cats and dogs 2 to 10 kg

   Partial energy requirement = _____ $\times \ 0.25 =$ _____ kcal/d from dextrose

   Partial energy requirement = _____ $\times \ 0.25 =$ _____ kcal/d amino acids

   Partial energy requirement = _____ $\times \ 0.50 =$ _____ kcal/d lipid

   b. Dogs 10 to 25 kg

   Partial energy requirement = _____ $\times \ 0.33 =$ _____ kcal/d from dextrose

   Partial energy requirement = _____ $\times \ 0.33 =$ _____ kcal/d amino acids

   Partial energy requirement = _____ $\times \ 0.33 =$ _____ kcal/d lipid

   c. Dogs greater than 25 kg

   Partial energy requirement = _____ $\times \ 0.50 =$ _____ kcal/d from dextrose

   Partial energy requirement = _____ $\times \ 0.25 =$ _____ kcal/d amino acids

   Partial energy requirement = _____ $\times \ 0.25 =$ _____ kcal/d lipid

2. Volumes of solutions required
   a. 5% dextrose solution = 0.17 kcal/mL

   _____ kcal from carbohydrate per 0.17 kcal = _____ mL/d

   b. 8.5% amino acid solution = 0.085 g/mL = 0.4 kcal/mL

   _____ kcal from protein per 0.4 kcal/mL = _____ mL/d

   c. 20% lipid solution = 2 kcal/mL

   _____ kcal from lipid per 2 kcal = _____ mL/d

   Total volume = _____ mL/d/24 h = _____ mL/h

---

a bleeding tendency are typically better candidates for either a PICC or peripheral catheter. Poor skin condition or disease as well as the presence of wounds at potential catheter sites may also affect choice of catheter location.

SUMMARY

Peri-surgical nutrition of veterinary patients is in its infancy with considerable research to be performed to help improve quality of life in our small animal patients. Clues from human immunonutrition may be starting places for investigation. Considerations for future investigations should include essential nutrients, the underlying disease process, therapeutic goals, and species (dog or cat). There are succinct guidelines for meeting caloric requirements enterally or parenterally. Planning for nutritional support before surgery takes place is likely to be beneficial to patient outcomes, particularly in patients with severe illness or who are already debilitated. Taking into account case history (anorexia), method of feeding, metabolic abnormalities, and possible immunonutrition should be part of a complete surgical nutritional plan.

REFERENCES

1. Alexander JW, Supp DM. Role of arginine and omega-3 fatty acids in wound healing and infection. Adv Wound Care 2014;3(11):682–90.
2. Chow O, Barbul A. Immunonutrition: role in wound healing and tissue regeneration. Adv Wound Care 2014;3(1):46–53.
3. Pierre JF, Heneghan AF, Lawson CM, et al. Pharmaconutrition review: physiological mechanisms. JPEN J Parenter Enteral Nutr 2013;37(5 Suppl):51S–65S.
4. Jones NE, Heyland DK. Pharmaconutrition: a new emerging paradigm. Curr Opin Gastroenterol 2008;24(2):215–22.
5. Stechmiller JK, Childress B, Cowan L. Arginine supplementation and wound healing. Nutr Clin Pract 2005;20(1):52–61. Available at: http://www.ncbi.nlm.nih.gov/pubmed/16207646. Accessed April 6, 2015.
6. Burns RA, Milner JA, Corbin JE. Arginine: an indispensable amino acid for mature dogs. J Nutr 1981;111(6):1020–4. Available at: http://www.ncbi.nlm.nih.gov/pubmed/7241223. Accessed April 6, 2015.
7. Ha YH, Milner JA, Corbin JE. Arginine requirements in immature dogs. J Nutr 1978;108(2):203–10. Available at: http://www.ncbi.nlm.nih.gov/pubmed/621576. Accessed April 6, 2015.
8. Morris JG, Rogers QR. Arginine: an essential amino acid for the cat. J Nutr 1978;108(12):1944–53. Available at: http://www.ncbi.nlm.nih.gov/pubmed/722344. Accessed April 6, 2015.
9. Santora R, Kozar RA. Molecular mechanisms of pharmaconutrients. J Surg Res 2010;161(2):288–94.
10. Bansal V, Ochoa JB. Arginine availability, arginase, and the immune response. Curr Opin Clin Nutr Metab Care 2003;6(2):223–8.
11. Curran JN, Winter DC, Bouchier-Hayes D. Biological fate and clinical implications of arginine metabolism in tissue healing. Wound Repair Regen 2006;14(4):376–86.
12. Akbarshahi H, Andersson B, Nordén M, et al. Perioperative nutrition in elective gastrointestinal surgery–potential for improvement? Dig Surg 2008;25(3):165–74.
13. Kalil AC, Sevransky JE, Myers DE, et al. Preclinical trial of l-arginine monotherapy alone or with N-acetylcysteine in septic shock. Crit Care Med 2006;34(11):2719–28.
14. Ogilvie GK, Fettman MJ, Mallinckrodt CH, et al. Effect of fish oil, arginine, and doxorubicin chemotherapy on remission and survival time for dogs with lymphoma: a double-blind, randomized placebo-controlled study. Cancer 2000;88(8):1916–28. Available at: http://www.ncbi.nlm.nih.gov/pubmed/10760770. Accessed April 6, 2015.
15. Schloerb PR. Immune-enhancing diets: products, components, and their rationales. JPEN J Parenter Enteral Nutr 2001;25(2 Suppl):S3–7. Available at: http://www.ncbi.nlm.nih.gov/pubmed/11288920. Accessed April 6, 2015.
16. Zulfikaroglu B, Zulfikaroglu E, Ozmen MM, et al. The effect of immunonutrition on bacterial translocation, and intestinal villus atrophy in experimental obstructive jaundice. Clin Nutr 2003;22(3):277–81. Available at: http://www.ncbi.nlm.nih.gov/pubmed/12765668. Accessed April 6, 2015.
17. Kallweit AR, Baird CH, Stutzman DK, et al. Glutamine prevents apoptosis in intestinal epithelial cells and induces differential protective pathways in heat and oxidant injury models. JPEN J Parenter Enteral Nutr 2012;36(5):551–5.
18. Braga M, Wischmeyer PE, Drover J, et al. Clinical evidence for pharmaconutrition in major elective surgery. JPEN J Parenter Enteral Nutr 2013;37(5 Suppl):66S–72S.

19. Marik PE, Zaloga GP. Immunonutrition in high-risk surgical patients: a systematic review and analysis of the literature. JPEN J Parenter Enteral Nutr 2010;34(4): 378–86.
20. Braga M. Perioperative immunonutrition and gut function. Curr Opin Clin Nutr Metab Care 2012;15(5):485–8.
21. Fritsche KL, Shahbazian LM, Feng C, et al. Dietary fish oil reduces survival and impairs bacterial clearance in C3H/Hen mice challenged with Listeria monocytogenes. Clin Sci (Lond) 1997;92(1):95–101. Available at: http://www.ncbi.nlm.nih.gov/pubmed/9038598. Accessed April 7, 2015.
22. Schwerbrock NM, Karlsson EA, Shi Q, et al. Fish oil-fed mice have impaired resistance to influenza infection. J Nutr 2009;139(8):1588–94.
23. Waitzberg DL, Saito H, Plank LD, et al. Postsurgical infections are reduced with specialized nutrition support. World J Surg 2006;30(8):1592–604.
24. Braga M, Gianotti L, Vignali A, et al. Preoperative oral arginine and n-3 fatty acid supplementation improves the immunometabolic host response and outcome after colorectal resection for cancer. Surgery 2002;132(5):805–14.
25. Drover JW, Dhaliwal R, Weitzel L, et al. Perioperative use of arginine-supplemented diets: a systematic review of the evidence. J Am Coll Surg 2011;212(3):385–99, 399.e1.
26. Giger U, Büchler M, Farhadi J, et al. Preoperative immunonutrition suppresses perioperative inflammatory response in patients with major abdominal surgery—a randomized controlled pilot study. Ann Surg Oncol 2007;14(10):2798–806.
27. Stableforth WD, Thomas S, Lewis SJ. A systematic review of the role of immunonutrition in patients undergoing surgery for head and neck cancer. Int J Oral Maxillofac Surg 2009;38(2):103–10.
28. Tepaske R, Velthuis H, Oudemans-van Straaten HM, et al. Effect of preoperative oral immune-enhancing nutritional supplement on patients at high risk of infection after cardiac surgery: a randomised placebo-controlled trial. Lancet 2001; 358(9283):696–701. Available at: http://www.ncbi.nlm.nih.gov/pubmed/11551575. Accessed April 6, 2015.
29. Vidal-Casariego A, Calleja-Fernández A, Villar-Taibo R, et al. Efficacy of arginine-enriched enteral formulas in the reduction of surgical complications in head and neck cancer: a systematic review and meta-analysis. Clin Nutr 2014;33(6):951–7.
30. Heyland DK, Novak F, Drover JW, et al. Should immunonutrition become routine in critically ill patients? A systematic review of the evidence. JAMA 2001;286(8): 944–53. Available at: http://www.ncbi.nlm.nih.gov/pubmed/11509059. Accessed April 6, 2015.
31. Leandro-Merhi VA, de Aquino JL. Determinants of malnutrition and post-operative complications in hospitalized surgical patients. J Health Popul Nutr 2014;32(3): 400–10. Available at: http://www.pubmedcentral.nih.gov/articlerender.fcgi?artid=4221446&tool=pmcentrez&rendertype=abstract. Accessed April 6, 2015.
32. Blattner RJ. Herpangina. J Pediatr 1951;39(5):635–7. Available at: http://www.ncbi.nlm.nih.gov/pubmed/14889409. Accessed April 6, 2015.
33. Marimuthu K, Varadhan KK, Ljungqvist O, et al. A meta-analysis of the effect of combinations of immune modulating nutrients on outcome in patients undergoing major open gastrointestinal surgery. Ann Surg 2012;255(6):1060–8.
34. Cerantola Y, Hübner M, Grass F, et al. Immunonutrition in gastrointestinal surgery. Br J Surg 2011;98(1):37–48.
35. Zhang Y, Gu Y, Guo T, et al. Perioperative immunonutrition for gastrointestinal cancer: a systematic review of randomized controlled trials. Surg Oncol 2012; 21(2):e87–95.

36. De Assis MC, Silveira CR, Beghetto MG, et al. Is duration of postoperative fasting associated with infection and prolonged length of stay in surgical patients? Nutr Hosp 2014;30(4):919–26.

37. Heyland DK, Dhaliwal R, Drover JW, et al. Canadian clinical practice guidelines for nutrition support in mechanically ventilated, critically ill adult patients. JPEN J Parenter Enteral Nutr 2003;27(5):355–73. Available at: http://www.ncbi.nlm.nih.gov/pubmed/12971736. Accessed April 6, 2015.

38. Manzanares W, Dhaliwal R, Jurewitsch B, et al. Parenteral fish oil lipid emulsions in the critically ill: a systematic review and meta-analysis. JPEN J Parenter Enteral Nutr 2014;38(1):20–8.

39. Montejo JC, Zarazaga A, López-Martínez J, et al. Immunonutrition in the intensive care unit. A systematic review and consensus statement. Clin Nutr 2003;22(3):221–33. Available at: http://www.ncbi.nlm.nih.gov/pubmed/12765660. Accessed April 6, 2015.

40. Rice TW. Immunonutrition in critical illness: limited benefit, potential harm. JAMA 2014;312(5):490–1.

41. Marik PE, Zaloga GP. Immunonutrition in critically ill patients: a systematic review and analysis of the literature. Intensive Care Med 2008;34(11):1980–90.

42. Bower RH, Cerra FB, Bershadsky B, et al. Early enteral administration of a formula (Impact) supplemented with arginine, nucleotides, and fish oil in intensive care unit patients: results of a multicenter, prospective, randomized, clinical trial. Crit Care Med 1995;23(3):436–49. Available at: http://www.ncbi.nlm.nih.gov/pubmed/7874893. Accessed April 6, 2015.

43. Heys SD, Walker LG, Smith I, et al. Enteral nutritional supplementation with key nutrients in patients with critical illness and cancer: a meta-analysis of randomized controlled clinical trials. Ann Surg 1999;229(4):467–77. Available at: http://www.pubmedcentral.nih.gov/articlerender.fcgi?artid=1191731&tool=pmcentrez&rendertype=abstract. Accessed March 13, 2015.

44. Pontes-Arruda A, Martins LF, de Lima SM, et al. Enteral nutrition with eicosapentaenoic acid, γ-linolenic acid and antioxidants in the early treatment of sepsis: results from a multicenter, prospective, randomized, double-blinded, controlled study: the INTERSEPT study. Crit Care 2011;15(3):R144.

45. Pontes-Arruda A, Demichele S, Seth A, et al. The use of an inflammation-modulating diet in patients with acute lung injury or acute respiratory distress syndrome: a meta-analysis of outcome data. JPEN J Parenter Enteral Nutr 2008;32(6):596–605.

46. Rice TW. Enteral omega-3 fatty acid, γ-linolenic acid, and antioxidant supplementation in acute lung injury. JAMA 2011;306(14):1574.

47. Mooney MA, Vaughn DM, Reinhart GA, et al. Evaluation of the effects of omega-3 fatty acid-containing diets on the inflammatory stage of wound healing in dogs. Am J Vet Res 1998;59(7):859–63. Available at: http://www.ncbi.nlm.nih.gov/pubmed/9659552. Accessed April 6, 2015.

48. Chan DL, Rozanski EA, Freeman LM. Relationship among plasma amino acids, C-reactive protein, illness severity, and outcome in critically ill dogs. J Vet Intern Med 2009;23(3):559–63.

49. Plumb D. Plumb's veterinary drug handbook. 7th edition. Stockholm (WI): PharmaVet Inc; 2011.

50. Long JP, Greco SC. The effect of propofol administered intravenously on appetite stimulation in dogs. Contemp Top Lab Anim Sci 2000;39(6):43–6. Available at: http://www.ncbi.nlm.nih.gov/pubmed/11487252. Accessed April 6, 2015.

51. Quimby JM, Gustafson DL, Samber BJ, et al. Studies on the pharmacokinetics and pharmacodynamics of mirtazapine in healthy young cats. J Vet Pharmacol Ther 2011;34(4):388–96.
52. Eirmann L, Michel K. Enteral nutrition. In: Silverstein D, Hopper K, editors. Small animal critical care medicine. 2nd edition. St Louis (MO): Elsevier Saunders; 2015. p. 681–6.
53. Larsen J. Enteral nutrition and tube feeding. In: Fascetti A, Delaney S, editors. Applied veterinary clinical nutrition. West Sussex (United Kingdom): Wiley Blackwell; 2012. p. 329–52.
54. Delaney SJ. Management of anorexia in dogs and cats. Vet Clin North Am Small Anim Pract 2006;36(6):1243–9, vi.
55. Remillard R, Saker K. Critical care nutrition and enteral-assisted feeding. In: Hand M, Thatcher C, Remillard R, et al, editors. Small animal clinical nutrition. 5th edition. Topeka (KS): Mark Morris Institute; 2010. p. 477–91.
56. Dunn LT. Raised intracranial pressure. J Neurol Neurosurg Psychiatry 2002; 73(90001):i23–7.
57. Davidson J. Feeding tubes. In: Tobias K, Johnston S, editors. Veterinary surgery: small animal. St Louis (MO): Elsevier Saunders; 2012. p. 1974–90.
58. Willard MD, Seim HB. Nutritional management of the surgical patient. In: Fossum T, editor. Small animal surgery. 4th edition. St Louis (MO): Elsevier Mosby; 2013. p. 90–110.
59. Salinardi BJ, Harkin KR, Bulmer BJ, et al. Comparison of complications of percutaneous endoscopic versus surgically placed gastrostomy tubes in 42 dogs and 52 cats. J Am Anim Hosp Assoc 2006;42(1):51–6.
60. Jergens AE, Morrison JA, Miles KG, et al. Percutaneous endoscopic gastrojejunostomy tube placement in healthy dogs and cats. J Vet Intern Med 2007; 21(1):18–24. Available at: http://www.ncbi.nlm.nih.gov/pubmed/17338145. Accessed April 6, 2015.
61. Justin RB, Hohenhaus AE. Hypophosphatemia associated with enteral alimentation in cats. J Vet Intern Med 1995;9(4):228–33. Available at: http://www.ncbi.nlm.nih.gov/pubmed/8523319. Accessed April 6, 2015.
62. Chandler ML, Payne-James JJ. Prospective evaluation of a peripherally administered three-in-one parenteral nutrition product in dogs. J Small Anim Pract 2006; 47(9):518–23.
63. Chan DL, Freeman LM, Labato MA, et al. Retrospective evaluation of partial parenteral nutrition in dogs and cats. J Vet Intern Med 2002;16(4):440–5. Available at: http://www.ncbi.nlm.nih.gov/pubmed/12141306. Accessed April 6, 2015.
64. Pyle SC, Marks SL, Kass PH. Evaluation of complications and prognostic factors associated with administration of total parenteral nutrition in cats: 75 cases (1994-2001). J Am Vet Med Assoc 2004;225(2):242–50. Available at: http://www.ncbi.nlm.nih.gov/pubmed/15323381. Accessed April 6, 2015.
65. Crabb SE, Freeman LM, Chan DL, et al. Retrospective evaluation of total parenteral nutrition in cats: 40 cases (1991-2003). J Vet Emerg Crit Care 2006;16(s1):S21–6.
66. Lippert AC, Fulton RB, Parr AM. A retrospective study of the use of total parenteral nutrition in dogs and cats. J Vet Intern Med 1993;7(2):52–64. Available at: http://www.ncbi.nlm.nih.gov/pubmed/8501697. Accessed April 6, 2015.
67. Queau Y, Larsen JA, Kass PH, et al. Factors associated with adverse outcomes during parenteral nutrition administration in dogs and cats. J Vet Intern Med 2011;25(3):446–52.
68. Qin H-L, Su Z-D, Hu L-G, et al. Effect of early intrajejunal nutrition on pancreatic pathological features and gut barrier function in dogs with acute pancreatitis. Clin

Nutr 2002;21(6):469–73. Available at: http://www.ncbi.nlm.nih.gov/pubmed/ 12468366. Accessed April 6, 2015.

69. Chan D. Parenteral nutritional support. In: Ettinger S, Feldman E, editors. Textbook of veterinary internal medicine. 6th edition. St Louis (MO): Elsevier Saunders; 2005. p. 701–7.

70. Wakshlag J, Schoeffler GL, Russell DS, et al. Extravasation injury associated with parenteral nutrition in a cat with presumptive gastrinomas. J Vet Emerg Crit Care (San Antonio) 2011;21(4):375–81.

71. Mauldin GE, Reynolds AJ, Mauldin GN, et al. Nitrogen balance in clinically normal dogs receiving parenteral nutrition solutions. Am J Vet Res 2001;62(6):912–20. Available at: http://www.ncbi.nlm.nih.gov/pubmed/11400850. Accessed April 6, 2015.

72. Thomovsky EJ, Backus RC, Mann FA, et al. Effects of temperature and handling conditions on lipid emulsion stability in veterinary parenteral nutrition admixtures during simulated intravenous administration. Am J Vet Res 2008;69(5):652–8.

73. ASPEN Board of Directors and the Clinical Guidelines Task Force. Guidelines for the use of parenteral and enteral nutrition in adult and pediatric patients. JPEN J Parenter Enteral Nutr 2002;26(1 Suppl):1SA–138SA. Available at: http://www. ncbi.nlm.nih.gov/pubmed/11841046. Accessed April 6, 2015.

74. Sacks GD, Diggs BS, Hadjizacharia P, et al. Reducing the rate of catheter-associated bloodstream infections in a surgical intensive care unit using the Institute for Healthcare Improvement Central Line Bundle. Am J Surg 2014;207(6): 817–23.

Index

Note: Page numbers of article titles are in **boldface** type.

http://dx.doi.org/10.1016/S0195-5616(15)00103-5
0195-5616/15/$ – see front matter © 2015 Elsevier Inc. All rights reserved.

Moving?

Make sure your subscription moves with you!

To notify us of your new address, find your **Clinics Account Number** (located on your mailing label above your name), and contact customer service at:

Email: journalscustomerservice-usa@elsevier.com

800-654-2452 (subscribers in the U.S. & Canada)
314-447-8871 (subscribers outside of the U.S. & Canada)

Fax number: 314-447-8029

Elsevier Health Sciences Division
Subscription Customer Service
3251 Riverport Lane
Maryland Heights, MO 63043

*To ensure uninterrupted delivery of your subscription, please notify us at least 4 weeks in advance of move.

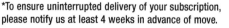

ELSEVIER

Printed and bound by CPI Group (UK) Ltd, Croydon, CR0 4YY

03/10/2024

01040492-0001